Tales of an Unorthodox Veterinarian

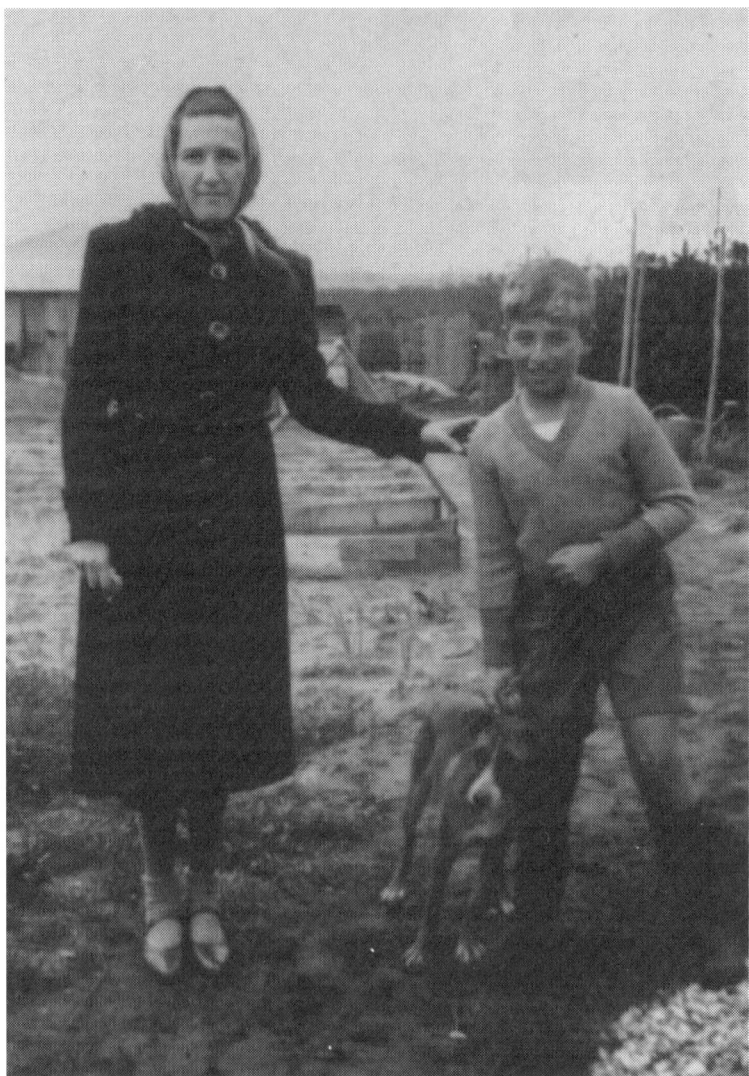

Tales of an Unorthodox Veterinarian

Dr. Gideon Sorokin

The Judah L. Magnes Museum, Berkeley, California

This book would have never been completed without the hundreds of hours of discussion and editing, and endless moral support offered by the following: my beloved wife, Cherie, the major contributor; Owen Phillips; my mother-in-law Holly Arpen; Mrs. Carol Castello, who assisted in editing portions of the book; Nelda Cassuto, who completed the final editing, and Jennifer Fisher, who provided comments and assisted with the typing of the manuscript. Thanks also to my sons Sam Sorokin and David Knowles.

Publication made possible, in part, by a grant from the Leona Shapiro Publication Fund

Published by the Judah L. Magnes Museum
2911 Russell St., Berkeley, California

Cover illustration: Anthony Dubovsky
Book design and production:
 San Rafael Design Group, Jon Goodchild

ISBN 0-942276-57-2

Printed in the United States of America

10 9 8 7 6 5 4 3 2 1

Contents

✳

Introduction

✳

This book was born of love of my Jewish heritage, and a desire to share with others the pride, joys, sorrows, and lessons I experienced as a child and young man.

The stories you are about to read did in fact occur. Some of the names and places have been changed in order to preserve the privacy of the living. This is not an autobiography, but rather a chain of true episodes from my life, all having one common denominator — animals.

Foreword

✳

There are so many sides to Gideon Sorokin that he makes a Rubik's cube appear easy to solve. I first met him ten years ago, shortly after he opened his animal hospital in Marin County, California; he later became my friend and employer.

This man must be related to a whirlwind. He gets up before the sun rises, calling people on the telephone to give instructions or tell them about a fantastic idea that occurred to him in the middle of the night. I am convinced he hardly ever sleeps. His briefcase—papers stuffed inside and many hanging out, notes to himself written on anything he can get his hands on, including paper bags—resembles a battlefield. And indeed the only thing he hasn't lost is his desire to achieve.

Gideon Sorokin is a person with a brilliant mind. He may be a trifle unpolished by American standards, but his interests and endeavors are so diverse that one cannot help but admire him. He sustains such a high level of energy that after spending an hour with him, one feels completely drained. Here is a man who never just enters into a project; he explodes into it, as if he had a rocket attached to his body. The word "moderation" isn't part of his vocabulary; nor is the word "impossible."

Gideon demands a great deal from people, but he has never asked me, either as friend or employee, to do anything that he himself wouldn't do. Despite his degrees and his profession, I have personally seen this man fix toilets, hammer nails, scrub floors, and single-handedly install an air conditioner where even the experts said it couldn't be done. He has no patience with incompetence and always expects everything to be done the day before yesterday. Gideon can have me climbing the walls, so frustrated I could strangle him. He can also make me laugh and feel better about myself than anyone I know.

Gideon was born February 9, 1930, to Jewish parents, in

Vienna. The family suffered for eight months under the Nazi regime, escaping in the fall of 1938, on the eve of World War II. As a child in Palestine, he worked selling fruit, and became an egg and chicken merchandiser while attending high school. During his high school years he studied Jewish literature, folklore and traditions in depth.

At fourteen, Gideon Sorokin became a member of the Haganah underground, helping to fight the British Mandate authorities and their discrimination against Jews in Palestine. With the creation of the state of Israel, he joined the Israeli Air Force. Gideon was in charge of security clearance for foreign pilots and volunteers who came to the aid of the struggling new state when it was being invaded by five other countries.

Gideon married at the age of twenty-one, and began his studies at the Hebrew University in Jerusalem. Later he went on to graduate as a doctor of veterinary medicine from the School of Veterinary Medicine in Pisa, Italy. Dr. Sorokin returned to southern Israel to practice Large Animal medicine in an area adjacent to the Gaza Strip. Later, he moved to the Upper Galilee, and worked in the border zones near Syria and Lebanon.

In 1961, Dr. Sorokin moved to Switzerland as an Assistant Professor at the University of Zurich. He arrived in the United States in 1962, and worked as a veterinarian for the United States Department of Agriculture in Montana, California, New York, Pennsylvania, and Alabama.

Dr. Sorokin presently lives and practices small animal medicine in Marin County, California. Well versed in seven languages, he lectures in the Middle East and around the world on the subject of veterinary medicine.

SANDRA CHARCHAF

I

Me and My Cat

✳

They called me Gidi and, like most children, I believed that I was very important, and that everything in the universe revolved around me. But the name I had been given did not seem at all impressive to me — not like "Nelson" or "Napoleon". It was my Papa's fault.

My Papa was the most stubborn man in all of Europe. While many Jewish families gave their children one Hebrew and one non-Hebrew name, my father, very proud of his heritage, insisted on two Hebrew names. Gidi was short for Gideon, portrayed in the Bible as a tough and determined leader in the fight for his people's survival. This name, I could live with. The other name, which I liked much less, was Yehuda (Judah), one of the twelve tribes of Israel. You can imagine that in a climate of not-so-subtle hatred of Jews, both of these were weighty names for a child to carry — especially in Vienna in 1937.

In my class at school I was one of only two known Jews . Though both Kretshi and I were good students, our teacher — the tall, blond Mr. Stecklmacher — tolerated our presence only because he had to under Austrian law. Even then, he only barely put up with us. I never understood why Mr. Stecklmacher hated us, but his sentiments were obvious. Every morning at roll call when he pronounced my name, our teacher assumed the hostile, wincing face of someone chewing on a piece of bone. And every day I stared straight into his eyes, defiant against his hatred.

In retrospect, I suppose that Mr. Stecklmacher had good reason to be uneasy about us. The Jews in his class were the best students, often winning all the awards, and he was obliged to report this "Jewish Problem" to the principal, Mr. Waldheim, at every teachers' meeting.

Sophisticated and well-attired, Mr. Waldheim played a game of diplomacy and courtesy at the teacher-parent meetings. "Your Gidi is certainly a successful student," he would tell my father. "He will someday make another Jewish doctor or lawyer" — insinuating that there were quite enough of us already. He would always follow the supposed compliment with something negative: "But, Mr. Sorokin, you are so fashionable. Can't you do something to make sure your son doesn't come to school dressed in yellow socks, green pants and a red shirt?" Even though I was just a shrimp of a child, I would have liked to punch Mr. Waldheim in the nose for tarnishing what was, to me, my impeccable image.

My Papa, in contrast, was a tall, well built and extremely well-dressed gentleman. His fifty immaculate suits and shirts and almost fifty pairs of shoes were kept ready every day by our maid, Hedwig. After admiring my father's good taste, Hedwig, like Mr. Waldheim, would tease me about the way I dressed, saying, "You take a shower every day, even when you are clean, but you can't even dress properly!" In the end I made up my mind to ignore her — indeed my father wasn't the only stubborn one in the family.

Hedwig was very devoted to our family. She was a hard worker and a good cook, and though I was jealous that she paid more attention to Papa than to me, I secretly liked her. When Hedwig heard Herr Sorokin approaching the front door, she always opened it and helped him take off his coat and hat. She would bow deeply and greet him with what seemed to me an exaggeratedly friendly "Good evening!"

Hedwig was a devout Catholic, and I suspect that one of the reasons she showed so much respect for my father was because he brought her a gift from the Holy Land every time he traveled there. During the course of the time she worked for us, Papa gave her an olive wood cross, a nativity scene, and the most important gift of all, a bottle labeled "Holy Water" from the Jordan River.

Toward my mother, Ella, I felt a tender love. She was slender, quiet, and sophisticated, and devoted to Papa and our family. I thought she was totally overshadowed by my strong-willed Papa, but she and I occasionally shared a secret smile when my father didn't quite get his way.

I remember that Papa, a fanatic for cleanliness, always insisted that Hedwig wear a wide head cap, so, God forbid, no hair of hers would ever fall into the soup. Well, one Sunday during the traditional family lunch, Hedwig brought in the three bowls of soup. As Papa raised the first spoon, to our amazement, we witnessed the sight of a five-inch-long hair draped around it. The hair was obviously Hedwig's. My Papa's fury erupted like a volcanic explosion. Hedwig cried and begged forgiveness for her terrible transgression. My mother weathered the storm stoically, showing no sign of a reaction, but as I sat quietly, trying hard not to laugh, I saw a brief smile cross her face.

My brother, Dov, nine years older than I, was not at home, for

Papa had shipped him off to an agricultural college in Palestine. I didn't really mind my brother's absence, for he would have taken center stage in our home. And though I don't remember anything specific about Dov from those days, it did always seem to me that Papa thought my brother was perfect.

Papa may have dressed like an aristocrat, but our home was no mansion. It was a rented apartment in the Goethe Hof, the largest apartment complex in Vienna. Papa, a very active and devoted Socialist, was granted a two-bedroom, second-floor apartment as a reward for his activism in the party. There was no doubt in my mind that we were lucky to live in this complex; our apartment boasted a fine view and a very good location. Built on the banks of the beautiful Old Danube, it was also modern, and included kindergartens, playgrounds and other facilities that children in Europe rarely had an opportunity to enjoy.

I was the only Jew on the junior swim team. We competed against the other Viennese Socialist housing complex, Karl Marx Hof. At one swim meet I became the youngest child ever to cross the Old Danube. This was the only sport in which I excelled, and indeed all of my athletic achievements after that swim were minor in comparison.

The day of my big swimming success has special significance for other reasons as well. For it was that evening that Minka, the most important member of my family, came into my life. On my return from the river, arriving at the door of our apartment, I nearly stepped on a scroungy, dirty cat. The animal looked into my eyes, asking for love. She was hungry and very weak. That day I was feeling strong and proud and needed to share my success with someone. It was the beginning of my love affair with Minka. I took the poor cat inside and washed her, despite violent protests from Hedwig, who was frightened of Papa's wrath in case Minka's hair got into the wrong place.

A month passed; Minka became healthy and strong, but most important of all, she became my real friend. Minka wasn't just a pet; she was my active companion. She followed me, as if to defend me from unknown enemies. She sat on top of my table to watch me study. I loved to watch her chase her tail. Her favorite activity was to try to steal Mom's wonderful *gefilte* fish. She always had a new plan of attack.

I can still vividly remember one Passover eve when Mom got up in the wee hours of the morning to cook a big batch of *gefilte* fish. Awakened by the heavenly smell from the boiling, spicy fish, I ventured into the kitchen. Minka, of course, was already there, pacing with anticipation. When the dish was done, Mom put the covered pot on the kitchen stool to cool off before Hedwig would put it in the icebox.

"Now, Gidi, you watch Minka to make sure she doesn't get into the fish," called Mom as she left for work. "You know how tricky she is!"

As soon as the door shut behind her, Minka ran straight to the kitchen. Quick as a wink, she jumped on the table above the stool and then jumped down hard on the heavy pot cover, kicking it sidewise. Before I caught up with her she had grabbed one of the balls of fish and scurried under the table to enjoy her feast. Miraculously, Hedwig hadn't heard the noise of the pot lid being knocked off! I quickly put the lid back on the pot, hoping no one would notice the theft. Fortunately for both Minka and me, nobody did.

Minka was both my cat and my buddy. She was the only living soul about whom I had no doubts or reservations whatsoever. Naturally, she slept in my bed on a pillow reserved especially for her. Often she snuggled under the blankets, warming up my body on a cold winter night. Her purring was an endless symphony that made me feel peaceful and content.

Growing up in our home, I felt as happy and fortunate as a child could be. I loved studying, my family, and my cat. Yet, perhaps, it was too perfect to last. For that infamous day, March 13, 1938, arrived and I would no longer be so lucky. Now, an eight-year-old kid doesn't understand a great deal about politics. Indeed, many adults never know or care a lot about politics either. But I tell you, everyone without exception gets scared when events unfold as they did in 1938.

My childhood ended on that night, when hundreds of German tanks roamed the streets of Vienna, and the skies filled with Junker planes whose engines rattled the windows of our home. In the streets crowds of Nazi sympathizers paraded, carrying banners of joy about the annexation of Austria to Germany, the greatness of Hitler, and the wickedness of the Jews. Among them I saw our principal, Mr. Waldheim, holding a banner that blamed the Jews for inflation, crime, and the promotion of another world war. Mr. Stecklmacher marched right behind him, doing just what his boss told him to.

If Mama was terrified of what the future would bring, I was confused. It was incomprehensible that I could be blamed for the world's problems. I had been a good boy. My teachers themselves had given me straight A's in school. How could they blame me for anything at all?

There were a few gunshots that night as some Socialists made a last stand against Hitler's Nazis, but it was to no avail. The Socialists were beaten up, some of them even killed. Most of those who resisted were sent to Dachau in Germany, the first known concentration camp for "troublemakers" — those who openly defied the new regime.

For the next two or three days Papa continued to go to the electro-technical supply store we owned. People seemed to be adjusting to the takeover. On the fourth day a neighbor called to warn us, "Ella, they are taking all the Jews to clean up the election slogans off the sidewalks of Vienna." Mom, Minka and I immediately locked the doors, pulled the shades and made no noise. A Gestapo agent knocked on the door so hard we were afraid it would be toppled. But he didn't break the door, and that day we were spared .

The next morning Mom took me to school as usual. I sat down and prepared my homework for inspection by Mr. Stecklmacher, but I had a strange premonition of something extraordinary to come. The usual knock and opening of the door announced the arrival of the teacher. Yet on this day, along with Mr. Stecklmacher came Mr. Waldheim. To our amazement, instead of civilian clothes, the principal wore an SA (Nazi Police) uniform with a swastika armband.

We all stood at attention. The two men had frightening expressions on their faces. The teacher ordered us to sit down. We did. Then Waldheim began screaming in an unnatural voice, almost an imitation of Hitler.

"From now on every morning all you children will stand at attention when I come in and with your right hand will salute and say, 'Heil Hitler.' I want you to practice this now!"

The class saluted, all except me and Kretshi. Mr. Waldheim then commanded all the students, "except the Jews," to sit down. When Peter Billig sat down, Waldheim told him to stand up again, saying, "Billig, you are Jewish too, because of your mother." To the three of us, he said, "You Jewish pigs, by decree of the Nuremberg laws, will no longer contaminate our children in the classrooms of Austria with your damaging behavior. Get your stuff and out you go!"

We were terrified at being kicked out of second grade with no warning. Peter, of course, was the most frightened and upset, because he had never known before that he or his mother were Jewish. He turned white and fainted on the floor. His neighbor, Sigmund, bent over and tried to comfort him.

"Let that Jewish pig pull himself together, Sigmund. Get back to your desk," Mr. Stecklmacher screamed. Sigmund was the only one who tried to help. The rest just looked on, some laughing, some silent and frightened.

I was scared too and couldn't hold back the tears, but the order to "get out" because we were "disrupting the class" enraged me. I took my school bag, walked up to where Mr. Stecklmacher and Mr. Waldheim stood and from all three feet of my height, looked up at them.

"I swear that someday you will pay for this," I said in a strange voice not really my own.

I looked into their stunned eyes as they were hit with my curse. Then I turned to Peter, helped him up, and all three of us walked out of the classroom, never to return. Many years later I found out that Stecklmacher never came back from the snowy Russian front and that Waldheim lost an arm and a leg to shrapnel facing the Jewish Brigade of the British Eighth Army on the front at Monte Cassino, Italy.

Peter and I walked home together, with me supporting him as we walked. He lived just one floor below us. Our mothers were not home and the empty rooms gave us a terrible feeling of desolation.

We were not the only ones who suffered that day. My Papa arrived later, bringing my mother from the hospital. She was in terrible shape and had bandages all over her hands. On her way home from taking me to school, she had gone to the grocery store to buy some food. The Hitlerites were waiting there and dragged her into forced labor. A contingent of Jewish women from the neighborhood had to scrub anti-German slogans off the walls and sidewalks. Papa was so furious when he found out that he had stormed out of his store shouting his opinion of the beast that had done this to his wife to all who could hear his voice.

When I told Papa about my experience at school, he took me in his arms and embraced me so hard that it was wonderful in its sadness. I felt his strength penetrate my body.

"Gidi," Papa said, "You are a hero, a real Sorokin. The Sorokins have always been proud fighters, sometimes against unbelievable odds. One day I will tell you the stories." His words were comforting. It felt good to be part of this family bond of strength, even though I didn't know exactly what he was talking about then.

For the next few days, Dr. Klinghoffer, our family doctor, came to visit my mother two or three times daily, mainly to change the bandages on her hands. She had constant pain that only heavy sedatives could control. Mom never talked much, but on the fourth day, while sipping tea with honey from a cup I held for her, she began to speak in a voice that seemed far away.

"My Gidi, what I am about to tell you is not really for children, who should be shielded from the horrors of this cruel world. But events have thrust you into adulthood prematurely, and I must tell you what is happening to us.

"When the SA [Nazi Police units] first caught me at the grocery store, they whipped me right there, screaming, 'That is what you deserve, Jewish lady pig, for not opening the door when we came to take you to clean the streets like we Austrians have learned to clean your Jewish dirt for ages!' Then they pushed me into a small van with nine other women I knew from our neighborhood. We were piled on the floor like lambs going to slaughter. We were all sobbing, fearing we would be raped or worse. The most panicky was Mrs. Billig, Peter's mother. She thought she would not be considered Jewish because she converted to Catholicism long before her Peter was born. In fact she had even displayed the swastika flag from her window, but it did her no good. She was with us, treated like any other Jew. I tell you, Gidi, with her screaming and crying, 'I am German. I love Germany. I love Hitler,' it was a terrible scene.

"The SA locked the doors and quiet settled over us in the stuffy van. Luckily the trip was short. We were pulled out onto the sidewalk of the neighborhood trolley station that had been painted with slogans. The Nazis put buckets of lye into our hands, with brushes and water but no gloves. They ordered us to scrub the paint, whipping us to work faster. The pain was unbelievable. We all screamed and cried, while a group of neighbors, some of whom we knew, stood by watching with amusement.

"Mrs. Billig, so tall, beautiful and muscular, carried on the worst. She felt that she was not Jewish and that they had no right to treat her that way. Well, she gestured to the SA man with her fist and he responded by whipping her and finally ripping her dress and underclothes, beating her with her own high heels. She started bleeding from her head and nose. She lost all reason, beating back at the SA man. The Nazi took his gun out of its holster and started shooting at her. We all fell to the ground. Mrs. Billig tried to escape, but fell in front of an oncoming streetcar. She was too weak and too slow to get out of the way. The car couldn't stop in time and ran over her, cutting off both her legs. There was blood everywhere. Mrs. Billig died before the ambulance arrived.

"We continued to work in misery, hoping to survive this ordeal. After the scene with Mrs. Billig, the neighbors and bystanders dispersed, leaving only the SA men guarding us. They would release us only when the street was clean. I must have ended up in the ambulance called for Mrs. Billig, because I fainted suddenly from the lye burns and my heart condition and I don't remember what happened until I woke up in the hospital.

"Gidi," she said, "I know how difficult this must be for you to understand. But I won't live long and I wanted you to hear the story."

Mom's story shocked me, and it reinforced my vague realization that someday soon I would lose her and would have to continue to live, painful as that might be. I guess death is never real to children until it strikes very close to home.

Mrs. Billig's death, of course, did strike home. Peter was now an orphan. He had lost his mother and his dignity with the realization that he was no longer part of the superior race. A few days after his mother's death his father abandoned him, seeking to escape the neighborhood and the shame of having contaminated his Aryan race with Jewish blood.

Papa took Peter into our home temporarily until a place could be found for him in the Jewish orphanage. Peter was very depressed about the loss of his parents and confused about his new Jewishness. I gave him one of my Star of David necklaces, but he didn't use it for some time. He wasn't ready. I let him play with Minka and she even slept one night on his bed. She was wonderful. She snuggled close to him and he wrapped his arm around her warm body, burying his face in her soft fur.

Weeks went by. We began to accept that things would just keep getting worse. We were gradually and systematically isolated from everything. The fact that we couldn't go to school was terrible for me. I couldn't understand what we had done wrong. Peter and I had been among the three best students in the class. Was it a crime to be smart, to study hard?

My boat and our small lot on the Old Danube shore were confiscated by the governor's office. Now Jews couldn't swim or mix in recreational activities with people of the superior race.

With my father's help, Peter and I began evening lessons about the Bible, Jewish history and the geography of Palestine. That was the place where my brother had gone and where, according to Papa, we should all go as soon as possible. He told me that in Palestine there were hundreds of miles of seashore and there would be better swimming than we ever had in Vienna. The schools would be better, and the teachers would certainly not make anti-Semitic remarks.

When we were sad, Peter and I played games. We pretended we were already in Palestine, doing all the wonderful things that we imagined kids did there, playing ball, swimming, fishing. It wasn't easy watching from the window as our whole class marched by dressed in colorful Hitler Jugend uniforms, singing their way to a fun outing on the shores of the Danube. But if we were cooped up, at least we were together and had Minka to keep us company. She was not just an animal; she was like a sister who radiated love and affection.

Minka became even more important when we read in the newspaper or heard on the radio that Jews would not be allowed to go to the movies, the theater or the zoo. These rules were incomprehensible to me. Next came the edict that no Aryan housekeeper could work for Jews anymore. That was really terrible for us. Since Hitler's annexation of Austria and especially since Mom's injuries, Hedwig had become an indispensable member of the family.

Hedwig was grieved by the injustice done to her employers, who had always been kind and generous to her. Sometimes, on my way to the bathroom at night, I would pass by her open door and see her studying the Jewish books we used in our home school. She even discussed the possibility of becoming Jewish because she said she was ashamed to be Aryan. It was amazing for me to hear this, since things were so terrible for Jews now. How could she even consider wanting to be Jewish?

The order for Hedwig to leave came in a registered letter, personally delivered by the know-it-all block commissar. This was the beginning of the end. Hedwig obediently packed, kissed us all good-bye and said she hoped to be with us again someday. We were all crying.

"Well, Gidi," Hedwig said, suddenly pulling herself together, "You'd better be a real man and help Mom with all the things she needs. And don't let the Nazis win." That last phrase meant so much to me. It became my motto for the next seven years.

Conditions grew worse. One evening around six o'clock Papa came home very agitated. He had a small cut on his forehead and his clothes were roughed up and full of paint. He gave me and Peter quick hugs and disappeared into my parents' bedroom. Peter and I heard a loud argument and I knew something was terribly wrong.

Half an hour later Mom and Papa reappeared in the living room. Papa put a packed suitcase near the door. Within a few minutes a taxi came and all of us were driven to the *Südbahnhof,* the Vienna railroad station from which trains left for Italy. I had only five minutes to tell Papa good-bye. Then he disappeared into the last train car. Tears streamed down my face; I was afraid I would never see him again.

On the way home from the station Mom told us why Papa had to leave so suddenly.

"Today the government issued an order that Jews who own businesses must nominate Aryan commissars to take charge of those businesses." They would, for all practical purposes, become the new owners.

"This morning when your father went to the store, he found that the Nazi block commissar, the *Hauptmann,* had chosen Hans, who is just a teenager, to be our store commissar. He is only a stockboy and the least knowledgeable of our employees. But he is a Nazi Party member."

"You can imagine how your father felt! Somehow he managed to take it, but in the afternoon about ten Nazis in uniform entered, all staggering drunk, all laughing. They ordered Papa out in front of the store.

"Now you, Sorokin, Jew Pig," the *Hauptmann* said, "Write on your store window, 'Don't buy here. It's a Jewish pig store.'" Papa resisted for a minute, raising his voice in protest. But one of the men hit him with a whip, so he wrote with paint on the window as ordered. When he was through, they threw the rest of the paint at him. It got all over his clothes. They finally left, but promised to return to take him to Dachau to re-educate him.

"Now you know why he had to leave. Tonight he will go to Italy and then on to Palestine, where he'll be safe. When he can, he will send for us."

The next morning at dawn, a black-uniformed SS man came to take Papa to the concentration camp, but was disappointed to find that Papa had already left for Italy.

The house felt so empty with Papa gone. I missed him. I missed my school and my boat. My Mom was injured. Hedwig wasn't there to help anymore. I couldn't understand what was happening. Why was the adult world so cruel? My only support was Minka, who had become even closer to me, snuggling in my bed with her cuddly warm body. Sometimes I wished that, by some magic, I would be transformed into a cat and not suffer anymore. But in the real world, there was no magic, only the harsh reality of the present.

One night there was a knock at the door. My mother feared it was the Gestapo, but it was Mr. Billig, Peter's father. He was bundled up so that he was unrecognizable. He looked terrible; pale, skinny, unshaven and neglected. In the past, he had always been admired for his elegant appearance. Now it was all gone. The violent death of his Jewish wife, whom he had loved so much, combined with his disgraceful flight had ruined him.

He did not even attend the burial of his own wife in the Jewish cemetery. Jews couldn't be buried in the general cemetery anymore, so that the eternal resting place of the Viennese Christian citizenry would not be contaminated.

Mr. Billig told Mom that he had come to pick up Peter and take him away to someplace where no one would know the shame of his father's transgression in marrying a Jew, or of the Jewish blood flowing in Peter's veins. It was ironic, a non-Jewish Austrian suffering so much from the Nuremberg laws!

Peter was awakened. He barely recognized his dad. When he heard that it was time to leave he started crying. Peter knew that we would never see each other again. I also knew I was losing a friend forever. Peter and I had grown very close in the last few weeks, as we had suddenly and reluctantly faced a common destiny. Peter and his dad left, carrying a shabby blue suitcase, and disappeared forever into the dark Vienna night of 1938.

I felt so lonely the next morning with just the three of us left: Mom, Minka and me. I lay in bed wondering, "What now?" No school. No one to play with but Minka. Mom could barely open a door with her burned hands. No Papa.

Finally Mom woke up that morning and came into my room. She was wearing a beautiful satin nightdress, the kind Papa always liked. The long sleeves of the gown hid her burned hands. To me, she was still the most beautiful and affectionate mother, although she was now weaker and paler than before. She gave me one of her warmest hugs, then positioned herself in front of me.

"Well, Gidi, there is no use hiding anything," she said, in a low whisper. "We are in deep trouble and I believe things will now get much worse each day. It will take Papa a few months to get us the visas to leave to go to Palestine.

"In the meantime, there is some good news. I have finally found a space for you at the Jewish orphanage. I just can't care for you anymore and you need a good school where you can learn. Without Nazi teachers."

I tried to be strong and not show Mom how terrified I was by her words, but I couldn't. I started to cry so hard that even today I am ashamed of it.

"I'm going to lose my home, my Minka and you, Mom! Be an orphan even though I am not one! I want to stay with you!"

Mom, however, explained to me that because Papa had been on the board of directors of the orphanage, she was able to arrange for Minka to go with me. She assured me it would all be temporary, just until we got our visas to Palestine.

The next day I left the Goethe Hof, the Old Danube and the little neighborhood I loved, for good. The fact that Mom had arranged for Minka to stay with me in the orphanage was a great source of consolation. Minka was the last vestige of my crumbling childhood.

The green taxi arrived. Its engine squeaked and moaned in a music that was appropriate to my sadness. With Minka frightened and tucked inside my coat, we were driven far across town to the orphanage. Minka stuck her little head out of my coat from time to time, asking with a quiet meow "Where are we going?"

We entered the *Waisenhaus der Wiener Jüdischen Kultusgemeinde*, the Jewish orphanage, after being checked at the gate by two very arrogant Austrian SA men. Besides checking my luggage they wanted to know whether my missing father was one of the Jewish troublemakers being punished at the Dachau concentration camp. When they heard that Papa was in Palestine, they commented, "Good! There the Jews will cheat each other and not spread their diseases to us."

My mother ignored their comments. I was very scared and felt helpless, though in my imagination I plotted ways to avenge the defamation of my father.

We entered the orphanage, a massive grey building, which had once been a retreat for high government officials during the Austrian Empire. As Austria shrank from a world empire to a small European country, the building had become a surplus. The manager, Mr. Moses Neuman, received us in his office. I liked him from the start, mainly because he had the same name as my grandfather, my mother's father who had died two years earlier. His Franz Joseph beard, genuine smile and above all his affection for Minka, made us instant friends.

The door of my room was close to his office and Minka quickly made the office her home when I was in school. She used to spend her time sitting on the file cabinet, her watchtower for keeping an eye on Mr. Neuman while he worked. I sometimes think Minka knew that Mr. Neuman was the equivalent of a Jewish saint.

According to Jewish tradition, God secretly sent thirty-six *Lamed Vav Zadikim* (righteous men whose identity no one knew) to the world to do exceptional deeds and experience personal sacrifices beyond the call of duty. In my mind, Mr. Neuman had to have been one of the thirty-six. He became the father of all of us fatherless children. He always tried to cheer us up, and when we cried, which was often, he took us in his lap and hugged us with a warmth that penetrated each of us. I think we cried sometimes just to be hugged by Mr. Neuman.

My roommate at the orphanage was Herbert. He was about the same age as I, but his father was in a concentration camp for being one of the outspoken socialists of Red Vienna who had tried to make a last stand when the Nazis took over. He was also Jewish. Herbert had nightmares about his father being beaten and forced to stand for hours in the snowy winter cold. Herbert saw him in his dreams, with his head shaven, getting more and more skinny. There was rarely a night that Minka and I weren't awakened by Herbert screaming. I was chosen to be Herbert's big brother, even though I was younger. Minka, too, tried to comfort him. Sometimes she would crawl into his bed, snuggling up against him to offer solace. Sometimes I wondered what was in the soul of Minka that made her better than lots of humans. Had she once been human herself?

The orphanage school was wonderful. All the boys were motivated to learn. It seems to me that we learned more in a day than I had learned at my old school in a week. In addition, we were taught Jewish history and religion. We learned about heroes like Moses, Joshua, and my name-sake, Gideon. Heroes were so important to us at that time, when we felt so low, helpless and frightened.

The number of children living there grew beyond the orphanage's capacity. Soon there was a third boy in our room. He had to sleep on the floor on a mattress, but that was better than the street where he had been sleeping. The quality of the food also got worse, but no one ever went hungry.

My Mom visited me only once a week, on Sundays. She tried to hide the troubles she was experiencing alone, and the pain of being bossed around by our former stockboy, who was very abusive in his new capacity as commissar. She kept encouraging me with talk of our departure to Palestine, although sometimes I doubted that we would ever be with Papa again. My mother seemed so frail. I knew she was suffering.

Two months later, though it seemed much longer, our redemption was announced by a phone call. We had gotten the passports and visas to Palestine via Italy! That day Mom put a sign on our store after all the employees were gone, including Hans. It said, "Closed for two weeks vacation." She sent the keys, with a thank you, to our largest creditor, so no one could say the Sorokins didn't pay their bills; the remaining mer-chandise and stock in the store was worth well more than our debts.

The message of our visas was delivered to me by Mr. Neuman, in private in his office. I still remember how hard I cried. Soon I was sitting on his lap, engulfed in his arms. He started to cry too. I had never seen a grown man cry before. I still don't know if they were tears of joy that Minka and I would soon be free, or tears of farewell, knowing that he and the rest of the kids would be remaining and would possibly suffer a terrible fate.

"Gidi," Mr. Neuman said, when he regained control of his emotions, "When you and your Mama arrive in the Holy Land, the land of our ancestors, promise to visit the Western Wall in Jerusalem and write on a piece of paper a prayer for all of us stranded here. Put it in the cracks for God to see. Perhaps He will save us."

On the last night I stayed at the orphanage we lit a candelabra, and although it wasn't Hanukkah, we all sang our hearts out. At the end we sang the *Hatikvah,* the song of hope for freedom in our own land. Suddenly, all the kids tried to touch me, as if to catch hold of my freedom for themselves. The tears flowed from every child's eyes, our destinies unknown but somehow bound together.

The next afternoon Mom came in a green taxi loaded with some of our belongings. She thanked Mr. Neuman for all he had done, giving him the *mezuzah* — the tiny metal container of the Ten Commandments that is placed on the main door of Jewish home — from our apartment. Mr. Neuman gave me a final hug. I would never see him again. Years later I found out that he died with his orphans at Auschwitz; his love and kindness stay with me to this day.

We got in our car, Minka in a pillowcase tucked inside my coat. At the gate the same policemen were waiting. This time they were even more abusive, hinting that Hitler would not allow us to leave because Jews were always stealing from Germans and must be punished. Only the intervention of the driver saved us.

We arrived at the *Südbahnhof,* the main station for southern destinations. Mom paid the driver, giving him a substantial tip for his help with the police. The driver said, "We will miss you, generous lady. Remember, not all Austrians hate Jews."

The porter took us to the train that went nightly from Vienna to Trieste, Italy. The train was full, but we were able to secure seats in second class. Jews could no longer travel first class. That night, at exactly ten o'clock, we heard the final whistle. Mom let out a sigh of relief at being able to leave Austria legally, but there were tears in her eyes. I hugged her, carefully, because her hands were not yet healed.

"Why are you crying?" I asked.

"Gidi," she responded, "Vienna was the place where I was born, grew up, and was educated. It was there that I fell in love with your Papa, bore you children and buried your grandfather. It is my home and we leave it never to return."

She was right; she never saw Vienna again.

The train operator sounded the double whistle to let all concerned know that we were on our way. I let Minka out of the bag. She was thirsty and gladly drank a few laps out of a glass of water. Soon she was the center of attention in our car — it wasn't everyday that cats go from Vienna to Italy. Minka sat next to me, purring and dozing, feeling somewhat safe in this strange place that moved with clickety-clack sounds. Passengers befriended her with offerings of cheese and salami, or leftovers from their sandwiches. Minka tasted some of everything.

Only one man stared at her with hostility. Later I saw that he wore a swastika on his tie pin and lapel. Maybe that explained it, but it still puzzled me. What could anyone, even a Nazi, find wrong with my Minka?

Hours passed uneventfully; the monotonous click-clack of the rails grew on us. My mother, however, remained very tense, hardly talking to any of the other passengers. Her hands were still stiff and sore and still oozing. But I felt better for the first time in months, as I liked talking to the other kids and adults on the train.

We were the only identifiable Jews on the car, though I thought one old bearded man might have been Jewish also. As we approached the border in the wee hours of the morning, the train conductor passed through all compartments of the train, announcing that passport control would commence, first by the Austrians and then by the Italians. Mom pulled out our passport, stamped with big letters, "Jews. Exit. No re-entry." I sat back quietly on the seat next to her, putting a reluctant Minka back into her pillowcase and under my coat.

Everyone got very quiet and nervous. Suddenly, the door opened and four SA men walked in. When our turn came they looked at my pale Mom, and asked for the passport. With great effort she handed it over. The policeman was tall and neatly dressed with a hard, mean look about him. Suddenly he approached me.

"Jew! What are you hiding under your coat?" I froze. My heart was going a mile a minute. In my terror I couldn't respond. He ripped my coat open and found Minka. He yanked her from me and started laughing, evil, sadistic laughter.

"Jewish cats have no visa and do not leave!"

He opened the window and threw Minka out of the moving train. I heard her terrible scream, part cat, part human, as she died under the wheels of the train.

I couldn't move. The horror immobilized me. The Austrian police moved on. I heard my mother whisper, "I hope that is the last Nazi I will ever see in my lifetime."

The policeman stopped at the next passenger, the old man with the beard. He also had "Jew. Exit. No re-entry" stamped on his passport.

"What you did to that child's cat was barbaric, shameful," the man said. The policeman raised his stick and hit him furiously. Blood gushed from the old man's head and mouth and he fell to the floor. No one moved. Fear and helplessness engulfed the train. But the man with the swastika on his lapel laughed harshly.

"That's what you get for opening your mouth, Jew pig."

Mom and I were frozen and numb.

The Austrian police moved on. I saw us speed by a sign that said, "Welcome to Italy." The Italian guards now moved through, checking passports. As soon as the Austrians left the car, one of the Italian border guards, with his funny feathered cap, moved quickly to the old man and helped him up. He brought him a towel and a glass of water, then turned to me and put his funny hat on my head.

"Some day you'll be a strong man and soldier, too, and will be able to avenge the wrong that was done to your cat and to your people. But, now, life must go on. You must be strong for your mother."

I composed myself, encouraged by the humanity of the Italian border guard. I got up, faced the window and the star studded sky. All at once I began to recite the Hebrew prayer for my dead cat, Minka. I first said the Kaddish and then the prayer, "Oh merciful God." Minka was closer to me than a human could have been.

The train continued to click-clack as before. But it's refrain was mournful now, echoing what I felt from my heart for Minka and her brutal death.

I believe in heaven, and I am sure that Minka is there.

II

A Donkey Of My Own

*

The train ambled southward into Italy, towards Trieste. The memory of the German border guards and Minka's screams were fresh in my mind, but the lulling movement of the train had a sedative effect. I dozed in between stops. At one of those stations, I got enough nerve to go outside to see if I could see any trace of Minka on the train wheels. But Mom called me back, afraid I might get lost in the crowd. "Gidi, don't you dare leave my side!" my mother scolded. "We have a long way to go before we reach Palestine. We are out of Austria, but not safe yet!"

I looked around the train car. Most everyone was asleep. At every stop, more and more Italians had boarded on their way to work in Trieste. It scared me that Mom didn't think we were safe. The Italians seemed so pleasant, and no one seemed to even notice us, except for occasional glances at my mother's bandaged hands. After her admonition I sat back in my seat watching everyone who entered the car for signs of trouble.

As we got closer to Trieste and no one but cheerful Italians entered our car, I began to relax again. I occupied myself listening in wonder to the beautiful Italian language, trying to catch the meaning of a word here and there. Suddenly it dawned on me that I would have to speak Hebrew when we reached Palestine. Although I knew a few words from prayers and songs, I began to worry about how I would be able to communicate with the other children. I wanted to ask Mom, but she still seemed so worried and tired, so I kept my anxious thoughts to myself.

What would Palestine be like, I wondered? I tried to remember everything Papa had ever told me about our pardess , the orange grove his family owned in Palestine. I closed my eyes. Instantly I was surrounded by hundreds of sweet smelling orange trees, in neat rows; so many I couldn't even count them. And there was a little white house with a red roof standing just next to the orange grove. Next to the house, a camel and a donkey grazed. I knew the donkey was mine! Papa hadn't actually told me what the house was like, but I was sure it was white and looked like a little Swiss chalet I had seen pictured in books. And though he had never mentioned anything at all about a camel or donkey, I was just as certain about them.

I fell asleep and dreamt a mixed-up dream in which my Minka, the store in Vienna, my grandfather's old-fashioned soda fountain, and our little rowboat on the Old Danube were all transplanted to our orange grove in Palestine, waiting for me with Papa, who I knew would meet us at the dock wearing his best suit and hat, and shiny black boots.

The sun shone brightly by the time the train pulled into the main station in Trieste. We were struggling with our luggage on the platform when out of nowhere a smiling lady with a big Red Cross cap and arm-band appeared. "Do you need help?" she asked, first in Italian and then, realizing we didn't understand, in German. "Are you Jewish refugees? Let me explain. This train now brings a constant stream of refugees, many of them brought out of concentration camps by a variety of means. Mostly Jewish, of course, but some are non-Jewish socialists while others were just people considered troublemakers by the Germans. I tell you, I don't know what this world is coming to."

When she stopped to take a breath, I piped up, "Yes, yes! Look what they did to my Mom's hands. She can't carry anything because of the pain. They beat up my Dad, too. He escaped and we are finally going to join him in Palestine!"

"You are lucky," she exclaimed, "if you have a visa for Palestine!"

"But we have to go without Minka," I said gravely, with tears welling up in my eyes. "They killed her. The border guard said she had no visa and he threw her out of the train!"

"Santo Gesù," exclaimed the Red Cross lady. "They threw someone out of the train? And killed her?"

"It was his cat," explained my mother. "He had her under his coat and the guard saw. . . ."

"Oh, my poor boy," sighed the Red Cross lady, stooping down and putting her arms around me. "I can't imagine! And to think there are Italians who want to follow those German beasts!" As she spoke, a group of black-shirted young men ran by us, shouting obscenities in our direction. I couldn't understand the words, but I recognized the hatred in their voices. Mom was right, we were not safe yet.

"Wait just a minute," the Red Cross lady said. "I will get someone to help you. Wait here with your luggage. Your mother can sit here on one of the suitcases. No one will bother you. I will be back with help in about twenty minutes."

I was a little afraid when she left, especially since I could still see the black-shirted boys out in the lobby. But they didn't return and true to her word, within twenty minutes the Red Cross lady came back with two men. My mother brightened immediately at the familiar sight of their formal dark suits and hats and aquiline noses. "Welcome to Trieste," they said in a language which sounded like Yiddish and Italian mixed together. I couldn't understand much, except that they appeared to be very reassuring to my mother.

"Come, Gidi," she said. "These are the Levi brothers. They have arranged a place for us to stay. They are part of a volunteer organization which helps people like us who are fleeing from the Nazis."

The room the Levis had arranged for us was small and two stories up in an old house, but it had a wonderful view of the port area where all the big boats docked. We shared a kitchen and bath with several other families, but it didn't matter. Everyone was friendly and the Levi brothers helped with everything! "Did you and Papa know them before?" I asked Mama, after she tucked me in bed that first night. "They are so nice to us!"

"No, Gidi," she responded. "They do this because they feel it's their duty to help. Your father and I would do the same for them if the situation were reversed. Remember, 'Kol Israel Chaverim ,' the people of Israel are all one family. I only hope they will not suffer as we have suffered, as others are suffering now. . . .

"It's good we are leaving, Gidi. I can smell war here in Europe. I can't wait until the *Galilea* comes and we sail!" The intensity of her voice frightened me, but I tried not to show it.

"It's all right, Mom. I'll take care of you! I can do it! You don't need to be afraid."

"Of course, my little one," she replied with a sigh. "Now go to sleep."

We spent ten days in Trieste, waiting for the *Galilea*. The Levis took us to their synagogue on Friday night. It was so different from what I was used to in Vienna. The *bimah* (pulpit) and altar were in the center and the seats were all around them. And the chants were so melodic. "It's the Spanish and Arabic influence," explained my mother.

"Spanish!" I exclaimed. "Papa once told me that the Spanish persecuted Jews. Was it like it is today with the Germans?"

"Well, very similar, I'm afraid," was her response. "I guess there hasn't been much progress in the last four centuries."

It was a very solemn service, with lots of prayers to God to save His children of Israel from the storms of persecution sweeping the European continent.

And what about the Arabs? I wondered to myself as I listened to the services. Did they hate Jews too? I knew there were lots of Arabs in Palestine. Could it be that there would be just as much trouble in Palestine as we left behind? I wanted to ask Mom, but she was busy talking to the Levis and by the time we got home from the synagogue, I was too tired for conversation.

Our days were spent waiting and watching the horizon for signs of the *Galilea*. I played a little with some kids who lived nearby, and I found a little grey kitty soon after we arrived and "adopted" her as my best friend. She didn't mind that I didn't speak Italian and seemed content to curl up next to me and sleep while I watched the shore with Mom. "Remember you can't take her with you," warned my Mom. "She belongs to someone else, and besides, the Captain wouldn't allow a cat at sea!"

Finally the day arrived. We spotted a big white ship with lots of portholes steaming into the harbor. "Look!" I cried. "It's the Galilea. You can see the name on the side!"

The Levi brothers appeared for the last time. "We will deliver you personally to the captain of the ship," they said. "We want to make sure you are both safely on board. *Hamazil adam echad keilu hizil et kol haolam* [He who saves even one human, it's as if he saves the whole world]."

"I want to be just like you when I grow up," I exclaimed as we shook hands and said good-bye on the ship's gangway.

The Levi brothers handed us over to the captain and explained our story. The captain was a tall, good-looking man who seemed genuinely pleased to have us on board. "We'll assign you to a cabin right by the dining room so your Mom won't have to use the stairs. You can sit at my table and if you are very good, I'll even let you steer the ship one day when the sea is calm."

"Steer the ship! Wow, would I love to do that. Anytime, captain!" I knew this was going to be a great trip.

I don't think I'll ever forget those six days on the *Galilea*. The sea was exceptionally calm. And because there were very few kids on board, I got lots of attention from the crew and other passengers. Our fellow travelers were all refugees headed for Palestine, mostly belonging to the middle class: well-to-do Jews from Austria, Germany, and Poland. Most had relatives or property in Palestine. A few had deposited huge sums of money with English banks to be used for enterprises in Palestine. This was just about the only legal way to get a visa. One or two passengers had bought visas either on the black market, or from sympathetic consulates of foreign countries. It seemed that everyone had a different story to tell about how difficult it had been to get a visa.

"But why is it so hard to get a visa?" I asked my mother. "Why can't everyone go to Palestine? I thought Papa told me the British promised Jews they could live there?"

"Well, this is a complicated political matter, Gidi. Your Papa was right, they did promise. But although the British have controlled Palestine since after the last war, there are many Arabs there. Now, because of the situation with the Germans, I guess the British are afraid that if they let too many Jews come, the Arab population may rebel or turn against them and start supporting the German war effort. Old promises sometimes get forgotten."

At the outset of the trip, the passengers as a group were subdued; the terrors of the past and fears of the unknown still overwhelmed us all. Even the flirtatiousness of the Italian waiters didn't seem to spark any interest among the girls.

Chess was a favorite pastime of many of the passengers and of the captain as well. I used to love to watch him play. Finally I got the nerve to tell him that my Papa had taught me to play and I was thrilled when he suggested a match. "If you win, I'll let you steer the ship for ten minutes, Gidi!"

"Wow! I don't think I'm good enough to beat you. But I sure want to steer the ship!" I prayed hard throughout the match that I would win, and miraculously, though undoubtedly through the intervention of the captain and not the Divine, I did.

"Well, little one. You are quite a player," said the captain. "I guess I'll have to make good on my promise now."

"Oh, oh," teased several of the passengers who had watched the match. "I bet we are in for a rough ride now! Are there any other ships in the vicinity? Better send out a warning to steer clear of us!"

"I'll be a good captain! You wait and see!" I responded, somewhat offended by their comments. I will never forget the sensation of steering that ship. Suddenly I seemed to be in control of my destiny. The terror and sadness of the past year dissolved. I was forging ahead to new lands and a new life!

Midway through our trip, the atmosphere among the passengers began to change. Fear was replaced by anticipation and excitement as we neared our destination. Four days of wonderful food — for some, the first really good food they had in months — also did wonders for the spirits. The fare was international, but with a heavy emphasis on Italian cuisine.

My favorite dish was spaghetti although I could never get the hang of how to twirl the strands around a big spoon. I preferred to slowly slurp the noodles into my mouth, one strand at a time. Of course, I made a real mess, getting so much sauce on my shirt that they nicknamed me "the spaghetti kid."

The last night on board, the captain announced a big show and asked the cooperation of volunteers among the passengers. The show turned out to be a mixture of everything: piano pieces, poetry readings, skits, dancing, and of course, singing. The waiters had taught me how to sing *"O sole mio,"* so I performed the song in fractured Italian, though with great gusto and to much applause. The show ended with an old Zionist song: "There where the cedars pierce the blue heavens, there where the land was soaked with the Maccabee's blood, that is the only fatherland we have. . . ." It brought tears to the eyes of the crowd, as we all thought of the land we were to become a part of tomorrow.

Everyone was up at dawn to watch the approach to the coastline. About half a kilometer from shore, the British immigration officials and police came on board; Tel Aviv had no deep water port, so the Galilea had to anchor well offshore. The British officers looked strange, wearing short pants, knee socks and shirts that were open at the neck. No ties, no jackets. The immigration officials had odd-looking blue/black flat top hats and the policemen wore tall black Persian lamb hats with a big silver badge in front. Even with their short pants and funny hats, they exuded a serious air of stern governmental authority. They took up positions near the gangway and everyone got in line to have their documents checked. We waited with apprehension; it seemed that everyone was being asked a lot of questions and the line moved very slowly. Finally, the captain came and took us up to the head of the line because of Mom's hands and generally poor physical condition.

"What happened to your hands? Why do you look so sick? Do you have tuberculosis?" barked the immigration official.

The captain interjected quickly. "No, no. It's just the aftereffect of the burns on her hands. The Nazis did this to her, can you imagine? How can educated Germans and Austrians do this sort of thing!"

The officer didn't appear very interested. As long as Mom didn't have tuberculosis and our papers were in order, his job was finished and he could move on to the next in line. He turned his attention to our documents for what seemed a very long time. "Welcome to Palestine," he stated at last after stamping and returning our documents. "*Eretz Israel* [the land of Israel]," said Mom in a quiet voice, as we turned to the policeman who was to escort us to the rowboat which would take us to the port.

The sea was choppy and I felt a little sick as we waited for the small boat to fill up so we could go to shore. "Don't worry," said Mom. "Soon we'll be with your Papa again and everything will be all right."

At last the boat was full, and a burly sailor expertly rowed us through the rough waters to the shore. Although it was early in the morning, it was already extremely hot and also very humid. The dock was crowded with people who were meeting the passengers, standing under big white umbrellas as a protection against the hot sun. I kept searching for Papa and my brother Dov among the crowd. When I finally spotted Papa, I could hardly believe my eyes! No three-piece suit or shiny black shoes! Instead, he was wearing a blue denim work-shirt and shorts! I scrambled out of the boat and ran ahead to him.

"Papa, Papa! We are here! Everything is fine! But, what happened to your clothes? Where is your suit?" I don't think I had ever seen him dressed in real work clothes, and I could only imagine that there must have been some disaster to make him go out in public dressed as he was.

"Why this is *Eretz Israel*, Gidi," he laughed and explained, as he hoisted me up in his arms and hugged me. "We're farmers now, not merchants. Besides, here even the big shots dress like this because of the climate. It's a whole new life. In fact, from now on I will call you Yehuda, your real first name. And so will everyone else. This is the Jewish home-land. You don't have to be ashamed to be called Yehuda. Remember, it's the name of the strongest tribe of Israel, origin of the house of King David.

"Here, let me reintroduce you to your brother whom you haven't seen for so long.... Dov, keep your eye on him while I go get your mother and arrange for the luggage." He entrusted me to Dov, who wore a British police uniform, except that he wore a big Australian military hat, typical of the Jewish Palestinian special forces.

"My, how you have grown, little one!" exclaimed Dov.

"Don't call me 'little'," I retorted.

"Now don't get testy," he replied. "There are some people here for you to meet again: the Rabinowitz family. You probably don't remember them. Papa and Mama helped them when they came from Russia and then paid their fare to Palestine. They have prepared a big lunch for all of us!"

"So, Yehuda Gideon Sorokin, welcome to Palestine!" exclaimed Mrs. Rabinowitz. "Your Papa and brother have been anxiously awaiting your arrival! We have a carriage for your mother and me and the luggage. You can come with us if you like, but perhaps you would like to walk through the city with the men?"

"Of course I'll walk!" I responded, standing up as straight as I could to make myself appear older. As we walked to the Rabinowitz's place, I was amazed at how few paved streets there were. And how few trees.

"These streets will be lined with trees before you know it," explained Papa. "There's a big project just getting started. The sand streets will soon be paved as well! Before long this 'hill of spring' [Tel Aviv] will be a big city!"

We entered a big plaza, where several movie houses were located. "At night, this is the heart of the city, Yehudale [little Yehuda]. Everyone comes here, even if they don't want to go to the movies. You live outdoors in Palestine."

Even at this early time of the morning the plaza was full of people. All Jews! Even the policemen were Jewish! It was an amazing feeling to be surrounded by Jews just going about their everyday life. I felt a tremendous sense of relief and security.

The Rabinowitz's apartment was very, very tiny. There was barely room for us all to fit in for lunch. But the food was wonderful and the atmosphere was comfortable and friendly. "I am going to like it here!" I thought. "This is a good place for Jews."

I confided my thoughts to Ida, the Rabinowitz's 18 year old daughter whose room I would share that night. "Well, you're right to a certain extent, Yehuda. But don't kid yourself that this is so safe a place. . . . There are thousands of Arabs in the city of Jaffa, a few streets from here. No Jews walk alone there at night. You wouldn't survive. The Arabs hate us and we have to fight for our survival here, too."

Ida's words terrified me. As I had not yet seen an Arab face to face, I had a hard time visualizing what it might be like if I was suddenly confronted by one on the street. I fell asleep wondering what I would do.

The next morning we left by bus for Ramatayim, our future home. Our luggage was piled on top of the bus with all the other luggage and cargo. The bus was crowded, but each of the four of us found a seat. We drove through endless orange groves, with millions of green oranges hanging from the trees. Herds of goats, some with big horns, grazed alongside the road; they made the driver very nervous because of their tendency to jump into the bus' path.

In the distance, I could see Arabs in long flowing robes moving in a caravan with a row of camels lead by a donkey and a rider. Every animal was loaded with enormous burlap sacks. The narrow asphalt road on which our bus traveled was only partially finished and twice we got stuck in the sand. Everyone had to get out and the men had to help the driver push the bus free. I worried silently about what would happen if a caravan suddenly appeared while the bus was trapped in the sand.

Finally, after a hot and sweaty two-hour trip, we arrived at the bus station in Ramatayim, which was actually a wooden shack with a small cashier's cage in the corner, protected by iron bars. "Not exactly like the *Bahnhof* in Vienna, eh, Yehudale?" said Papa as we picked out our luggage from the pile of suitcases and boxes still on the roof of the bus. "But at least there is no Nazi hatred here!"

"But what about the Arabs?" I asked.

"Oh, well, yes," he replied. "They are certainly part of our life and we have to learn to live in peace with each other. Sometimes that is difficult."

"They seem so different from us," I said, looking worried and thinking about the caravan I had seen that morning.

"Of course we are different!" he responded. "And we will both have to compromise a bit. They have learned a lot from us, and we can learn a lot from them, too. For instance, let me show you how much easier it is to carry heavy things the Arab way!" He then swung Mom's big suitcase onto the top of his head and balanced it there. "Come on, Yehudale. Try it yourself." With a little help from Dov I put my suitcase on my head, too. He was right. It was easier to carry this way. "See, my son. The Arabs have some good ideas. They have wonderful customs and are very hospitable too. You'll see."

We started off for home, looking like our own mini caravan. Papa led the way, holding one hand against the edge of Mom's big suitcase which he balanced on his head. Dov followed, holding Mom by the arm and carrying another suitcase with his free hand . I came last, a small suitcase on my head and struggling a bit to keep my balance in the deep sand. It must have been quite a sight.

Finally we arrived at a rusty gate below a big metal arch. "Here we are!" exclaimed Papa. The lock on the gate which led to our property was broken and the gate squeaked when Papa opened it. There were neat rows of very young fruit trees lining the way up to the house and two rows of grapevines which were flourishing. The air had a very sweet smell. At the end of the path stood a corrugated metal shack. It was really an orange packing house, consisting of one large room with no bathroom or running water. This was our new home. Not at all what I had imagined. I must have looked disappointed. "It's only temporary," smiled Papa. "one day we'll have a better house. At least here we are free and safe."

Almost as soon as we were inside, Dov kissed Mom and me goodbye and shook hands with Papa. "I've got to get back to work," he said, as he strode out of the door.

Mom was exhausted from the walk and immediately lay down on the only bed in the room. "Let your mother sleep a while, Yehudale. You help me unpack and fix lunch."

We had barely started on the task when I heard the rusty gate squeak again. "Someone is coming up the path," I called to Papa from the door.

"It's probably your Aunt Alice, Mom's sister. I'll bet she has brought your cousins, Chana and Jardena, with her, too. You'll like them!"

It was a tearful reunion for Mom and Aunt Alice who hadn't seen each other for at least 15 years. Chana and Jardena were teenagers. They spoke only a little German, having lived their entire lives in Palestine. We had a hard time communicating, but I was pleased that they didn't laugh when I tried out one or two of the few Hebrew words I knew. Aunt Alice immediately offered to teach me Hebrew. "After all, you'll be starting school in a few weeks. You'd better know some Hebrew before then!" And so it was arranged for me to start my lessons the very next day.

"Come on, Yehudale," called Papa after Alice and her daughters had left and Mom had fallen back to sleep. "Let me show you around the plantation. We've hardly had a chance to talk since you arrived. I want to know all about your experiences after I left. I know it must not have been easy, especially in the orphanage."

It was late afternoon as we set off for our walk through the orange grove. The air was heavy with humidity and the smell of citrus. Austria seemed very far away. It was wonderful to be with Papa again. I spilled out my heart and told him everything, including the story of Minka's death and my fears, especially after talking to Ida, that the Arabs may hate Jews in Palestine just as much as the Nazis hated them in Austria.

Papa put his big arms around me and gave me a warm hug. "I'm so very sorry about Minka, my son," he said in a quiet voice. "There is nothing I can do to bring her back. But you live in a new land now and will have a very different kind of life. I think you should have a special kind of pet, one that befits your changed situation. How would you like a donkey of your very own?"

"A donkey of my own! Oh, Papa! That would be wonderful. I always dreamt I would have a donkey if I ever came to Palestine."

"And so you shall. We'll go tomorrow before your Hebrew lesson and buy one from Sheik Abu Musa, who lives only about a kilometer from us."

"So close?" I asked with concern.

"Yes, the Arab village is just down the road from us. We can walk there and you'll ride home on your very own donkey. It will give you a chance to see that our Arab neighbors are very nice people, people we can live in peace with.

"Now it's getting late. Let's go home and have a quick supper and get you off to bed. I have a special bed for you, different from any you have ever had before! It's made of orange crates and woven grass and is called machzelet."

I was so tired by then, I could have fallen asleep on the bare floor. Indeed, I barely kept awake through dinner and Papa tucked me in as soon as we were through with our meal. I fell asleep instantly.

The next morning, Papa and I set out on foot for Abu Kishek, the nearest Arab village. "The Arabs you will meet today are really Bedouins, Yehudale. They used to be nomads, but now they camp permanently on this land. Except for the fact that they no longer wander through the deserts and mountains, they live pretty much as their ancestors did."

From a distance I could see large black tents set up seemingly at random on the little hills overlooking the green orange groves of Ramatayim. Herds of goats and sheep and small Arab cows grazed freely among the tents. As we approached the sheiks tent, scores of tan colored sleek dogs barked to announce our arrival. Suddenly, a tall dark-skinned man dressed in a flowing white robe with a dagger tucked into his large leather belt came out of the tent.

He addressed my father in a mixture of Arabic and Hebrew. *"Ya Adon, shu bidack* [what do you want, sir]?"

"I would like to speak to the sheik," my father replied in Hebrew. "Come in, please. The sheik will see you immediately. Your visit is an honor."

We entered the big dark tent. When my eyes adjusted to the darkness I could see a rotund old man sitting on large pillows covered with sheep and camel skins. He was dressed in the same white robes as the man who had greeted us wore, but he had a revolver in his belt and his white *kafia* (head scarf) was adorned with a golden braided agal (band). For me, it was like a scene from a Hollywood movie, only I was in it!

To my amazement, he got up and greeted us in Hebrew, which my father translated into German for my benefit. "You are welcome here. It is a great honor to have my neighbors in my humble home." Out of nowhere three veiled women appeared, bringing steaming cups of coffee and unusual cookies. I couldn't imagine how they had prepared this so quickly. Soon after, they brought out two little glasses of a clear liquid *arak* — for my Papa and the sheik to toast each other in peace and friendship.

"This is amazing," I thought to myself. "In Vienna there would never be so much ceremony over buying a donkey."

Twenty minutes elapsed before my Papa finally got around to the real subject of our visit. When he saw me getting a little impatient, he explained, "This is the Middle East, Yehuda. Things go slower here. Just be patient."

Finally my Papa got to the point. *"O ya achi* [my brother], I would like to buy a donkey from you for my son, to replace a cat he lost in Europe and loved very much." The sheik expressed surprise that anyone would want a donkey to replace a cat. "Well, my son loves animals. I thought he should have a pet that is also useful."

"I understand," replied the sheik with a slight smile. "For you, my neighbor, I am delighted to make a gift of one of our donkeys for your young son."

"Oh, no," exclaimed my father. "I couldn't accept such a gift. I would like to pay for the donkey."

"Well, if you insist. How about 20 Palestinian pounds?"

"With all respect, Sheik, I know donkeys are expensive, but I can only afford a 5-pound donkey for my son. . . ." This friendly haggling continued for about 10 more minutes until they finally settled on 10 pounds.

Papa pulled out the ten pounds and ceremoniously delivered them to the sheik. "I'll give you the best donkey I own, one that will be safe for your son to ride and useful as well."

"We are most honored by your graciousness," responded my Papa.

As we exited the tent, the donkey was already waiting for us. She was reddish-brown and the most beautiful little donkey I had ever seen. I reached up and hugged her and she reciprocated by licking my face and making a small braying sound. "Oh, thank you, Papa," I exclaimed. "Now I know I will be happy here. This donkey makes everything perfect again!"

Papa lifted me up on the donkey's big, broad back. "Hold on, Yehudale. You may think everything is perfect, but you still have a lot to learn in Palestine, including how to ride this donkey!"

From the corner of my eye I saw the Sheik's wives and children laughing at me as the donkey immediately took off in the wrong direction, almost throwing me off in the process. *"Dummkopf!"* I shouted at the donkey. "You are going the wrong way!"

"That's a good name for her," shouted Papa after me, laughing. After several false starts, I finally got her to take the right direction and Papa and I headed for home. I didn't even care that everyone had been laughing at me. I was truly happy for the first time in many months. I had my Papa back, a new and fascinating homeland, and a donkey of my very own!

III

Fatima, Fritz and Me

✳

T his story is rather short and, to tell the truth, I am not very proud to tell it. It is a story of revenge, and while revenge is sometimes understandable, it is never sweet or noble.

From the time I arrived in Palestine at the age of eight, I never really had a chance to play like other children. Besides going to school, I had to help care for my ailing mother and also help Papa with the orange grove. My brother Dov, who was in the Jewish Police Force, didn't live with us, but showed up twice a month to spend an hour with Mom and Papa, hand over part of his salary and disappear again. He zoomed in and out of our lives. Though in my parents' eyes he could do no wrong, from my perspective, he wasn't much help with the hard daily life in our new land.

The year was 1940, and the Germans, headed by Rommel, were at the gates of Egypt. The Arabs in Egypt were on the verge of switching their loyalties from the British to the Germans. The Jews of Palestine knew that it was a time of do or die. My brother told us that the British had been secretly training his unit for guerrilla warfare in case the regular British military forces abandoned Palestine for the mountains of Lebanon. My mother, whose health continued to deteriorate, was terrified by the thought of a German invasion. My father said he would rather die than experience another Nazi occupation. I was afraid, too.

The unfortunate day I will describe started like any other. I went to school, where I was still struggling with Hebrew and wasn't quite accepted by the other kids. After school I had a quick snack and then went to water our family's orange trees. I had to do this every three weeks during the summer and I used a big hoe to divert the water to each tree individually.

That day I was nervous because the news from the front was especially alarming and I kept wondering what I would do if the Germans suddenly appeared. As I watered the trees, I watched the road leading to the Arab village of Abu Kishek.

I had already learned a little Arabic, and had some Arab friends.

Among them was Fatima, one of Sheik Abu Musa's daughters. Looking back, I think she actually liked me. I let her cut grass for her donkey in our orange grove and I liked to watch her towering figure and bronzed features. I always used to wonder how she would look if she were not covered from head to toe in traditional black robes. Of course, I never told her that, for I did not want to offend her.

That day Fatima passed by the orange grove leading her grass-laden donkey; she was followed, as usual, by her mixed German shepherd dog. Now, I was reasonably friendly with Fritz, but not overly so. He was enormous, part black and part silver, and was always slobbering his great tongue hanging out of his mouth. It was also rumored that he liked to eat cats.

As she passed by me that day, Fatima stopped alongside the fence with a strange smile on her face. Suddenly she burst into laughter: "You Jews beware! By next week the Germans will be here and your grove will be mine and I'll be able to cut all the grass I want without having to ask you at all."

I was shocked and devastated. I had thought Fatima was my friend. I felt like the earth under me was shaking, but in reality, it was my anger welling up uncontrollably.

"No! I won't allow it!" I cried, "No more losses and humiliations! No more burned hands! No more Mrs. Billigs! No more Germans!.."

Again, I saw Minka flung from the train. All these thoughts churned through my mind. I seemed to gain supernatural strength. Jumping over the fence, I struck out blindly at Fatima with a wild orange tree branch. It was covered with short spines and made quite a deadly weapon.

I was hitting her as hard as I could, in my mind avenging my mother's pain, my Minka's death. She wasn't expecting such a fight from a ten year old kid. She fell to the ground, blood gushing from her mouth. I kept hitting and hitting. It was terrible, but I could not stop. I was feeling victorious, but then Fritz attacked me to save his mistress. The German shepherd tore into the flesh of my leg. I fell to the ground, blood pouring from my wound.

We lay next to each other for quite some time. Fritz was nervously circling around us, all bloodied up but still growling. Few people ever traveled on this road, but finally my father came by looking for me. As soon as he saw us, he ran to the nearest house and called an ambulance. We were both taken to the same hospital, lying side by side in deadly silence.

I was discharged within hours, though I had to return to the clinic to get a rabies shot every day for fourteen days. The dog bite took seven months to heal. Fatima remained in the hospital for three months, suffering from broken ribs and a lung injury. Her dog, Fritz, was shot.

I was called to the police station to make a report on the incident. The captain was very formal and cold, but next to him stood none other than my brother. Sometimes it helps to have connections. I told my story, repeated what Fatima said and described my own actions brought about by anger. The captain said something in English which I didn't understand, but my brother translated his words: "You know these Arabs can't be trusted for a minute. They are just itching to switch sides and start something with the Germans. They make my life miserable. I've got to protect them, be nice to them. And all the while they plot our overthrow. Personally, I think I prefer your little brother's direct approach!"

By appearances, I left triumphant, but in my heart I knew better.

There would be no winners in this battle: when we fell on that road, my neighbor and I, our blood was equally red, mixing together and soaking the soil of Palestine.

IV

The Not-So-Kosher
Merchant from the South

✳

A couple of years had passed since my landing at Tel Aviv on a chamsin day, a day of hot desert winds, as a Jewish refugee from cold Nazi Austria. In Palestine I was called a *Yeke,* an abbreviation for *Yehudi* kshe havana, which means "a German Jew who is slow and has a hard time understanding." I found this term quite insulting: nevertheless, like most of us young *Yekes,* I learned Hebrew quickly and soon established my position in the power structure at school.

One thing that really set me apart from the other kids was my private transportation, my donkey, Hyman. Other kids had to walk miles, so having a donkey to ride to school was like being chauffeured in a Rolls-Royce limousine.

Hyman was my second donkey and I bought him with money that I earned on my own. Let me explain. My father was an idealist and also very, very stubborn. For him, coming to Palestine was more than just an escape from the Nazis: it was a new beginning, a new way of life. To my father, Palestine was an agrarian state, and Jews who came there should be farmers. Unfortunately, he was basically a city person, a merchant of electrical equipment. He knew nothing about farming and, therefore, made very little money for our family, but he wouldn't give up on his ideal vision; he would be a farmer!

In 1940 times were very hard for farmers in Palestine, especially for citrus growers. All the shipping lines in the Mediterranean had been cut, so export was impossible. We labored all year round, watering the trees in the sweltering heat, pruning, plowing, and fertilizing. In the end, because there was no way to market the abundant crop, the bulk of the harvest would be dumped and buried in big trenches at the base of the sweet smelling trees where the fruit had grown. It was heartbreaking, especially because we knew there were people starving in war-torn Europe.

(Three years into the war, oranges were suddenly in demand again, as a chemist found an efficient way to use the oil extracted from the peels for the production of explosives badly needed for the Allied war effort. The pulp of the oranges was then fed to cattle. But let me go back to the story. . . .)

Because there was no money earned from the production of oranges when we first arrived in Palestine, my Papa concentrated on apples, pears, avocados, grapes and plums, fruits that were less plentiful than oranges and grapefruit. He also planted lots of tomatoes, peppers, celery and a few potatoes. Everyday, except on Sabbath, a big truck would stop at our gate and take five or ten boxes, whatever we had ready for sale, and deliver them, along with the boxes of the other local private farmers, to the Central Market in Tel Aviv for sale. But, despite the scarcity of food during wartime, sales profits were pretty poor. The driver and the market took a percentage, of course. The proceeds almost always fell short of what Papa expected. "Pilferage at the market," and "one of your boxes fell off the truck. . . ." were the most common reasons given, and though Papa grew suspicious, there didn't seem to be any better alternatives.

One day, quite by accident, I discovered that several of my school friends' mothers would be willing buyers of fruits, vegetables and eggs, if I would bring them to their homes.

"Do you have any extra products, Yehudale?" asked Mrs. Cohen one afternoon when I was describing some of my father's problems. "If so, bring me some. I'll pay you good money."

And so, at age nine, I became an entrepreneur, and I took my responsibility very seriously. Everyday after school I would take my two-wheeled wagon, pulled by little Dummkopf, to the village and sell eggs, fruits and vegetables to the housewives. I was also an important source for gossip. I was witty, up-to-date, and unthreatening to my lady customers, who loved stories, and they flocked to my little mobile stand for food and spicy news.

As my enterprise grew, I kept loading my little cart with more and more fruits and vegetables until it was almost too awkward and heavy for Dummkopf to pull. Finally, Papa suggested that we buy a bigger donkey. "It's too much for her, Yehudale. It's cruel to make her pull so big a load. If we buy another donkey you can hitch them together. Mischa next door has a beautiful donkey that he never uses for anything. I'll bet he would sell it to us cheap."

"Mischa has a donkey? I've never seen it."

"Sure. He keeps it on the other end of his pardess because there's better grazing there."

Mischa was our closest neighbor, an ardent communist who had immigrated from Russia to escape persecution as a Jew. He was only average size, but he had a high imposing forehead and long white hair. He looked a little like Ben Gurion, except he always wore red or black Russian peasant shirts with high round collars. He lived a very quiet life, but had fiery, intense eyes and a piercing look, particularly when he would start to talk politics. As we lived some distance from the village and there were no kids close by, I used to visit Mischa a lot, especially when I felt lonely. He was pretty gruff, but seemed to enjoy my company, even if I was a "young whippersnapper capitalist" whose specialty was making a buck while he waited for "justice and government by the Proletariat."

"Your Papa's right," he said sternly when I broached the subject of purchasing his donkey. "You work that poor little Dummkopf too hard. Besides she's not too bright. I've watched you struggle to get her going in the right direction."

"Yes," I admitted. "She's always had a little problem with that."

"What you need is a big, strong, male donkey. And you can afford it with all the money you rake in from the women of this town! I'll bring Hyman back with me tomorrow."

Hyman turned out to be a beautiful, mostly white donkey, with touches of brown here and there. He had big brown eyes and looked very intelligent and strong in comparison to Dummkopf. It was love at first sight for me.

"I'll take him. He's just what I need for my business," I said, full of self-importance. After only a little negotiation, Hyman was mine, paid for with my very own hard earned money.

With Hyman hitched to the wagon, I could really load it up, and we were able to travel much farther, too. Soon I expanded my territory to all the surrounding villages, where soon I became known as the hasocher *mehadarom,* the merchant from the South. More important, although I was only nine, my enterprise actually helped sustain the family. Naturally, it made me very proud and more than a little cocky!

We were quite poor, and the money I brought home was sorely needed. We were still living in the one room converted orange-packing house, with corrugated tin walls and roof and a dirt floor. Several months after our arrival, our furniture had miraculously arrived from Vienna on the *Galilea's* final trip to Palestine. (On her way back home she was sunk by the Allies.) Our precious furniture, however, was still in crates and stood on the porch only partially protected from the elements. My mother was still the only one who slept on a real bed. Papa and I had to be content with upside down orange crates which were covered with three layers of bamboo mats to soften their hardness.

Mom had never recuperated from the suffering she had endured under the Nazis in Austria. Her hands had second-degree burn lesions from the lye and her heart was severely weakened. Our housing conditions, with no heating in winter and no relief from the heat in summer, only made it worse for her.

Now, Mom had a wealthy brother named Karl in California. One day, a few years after our arrival in Palestine, she decided to write him about our plight. "I know he'll help us out," she said. "We'll be able to have a real house soon. We should hear form him any day now."

We used to talk about Uncle Karl a lot. "Any day now" became our refrain. But it was wartime and postal service abroad was very erratic and slow. In the meantime, we made do with what we had, and I continued to peddle our fruits and vegetables everyday after school.

When I was twelve, I started my second enterprise: the raising of rabbits. And again, Mischa was a big help to my capitalist schemes. As you may know, rabbits are not kosher, being rodents and not ruminants, and are therefore forbidden to devout Jews. For that reason, they weren't widely used for food. Mischa, however, had no dietary scruples and he used to raise rabbits for meat for himself. I used to help him feed them with fresh grass from the pardess whenever I would visit. I loved to hold them and pet them.

"Their fur is so soft, Mischa, it reminds me of my cat, Minka."

"Well, rabbits aren't too different from cats, Yehudale. Look here." He showed me a carcass of one of the rabbits he had just killed. "Looks just like a cat, doesn't it? The only real difference is in the leg joint."

"How do you know this, Mischa?" I asked, wondering if he had ever butchered cats.

To my relief, he just laughed. "Oh, I guess it's just common knowledge! Anyway, I don't know how I know it, I just do. When you get to be my age you don't remember these things."

One afternoon I stopped by Mischa's house on my way home from selling vegetables. "Still selling your fares with such fervor, Yehudale? Trying to get rich?"

"Hey, come on," I responded. "I'm just trying to help out Mom and Papa. Can I help it if I'm a natural salesman and all these housewives love me and the stories I have to tell when I come around?"

"I bet that you could sell ice cream to the Eskimos, Yehudale!"

"You think so? I wonder if I could sell some of your rabbits for meat? What do you think, Mischa? You know we have hardly any meat at all at home, and it's not just because Papa is a vegetarian. I bet it's the same everywhere."

"Of that I'm sure, given this war rationing," agreed Mischa. "But I'm not so sure you could sell rabbits to very many of your customers even so. Besides, I have no interest in raising more rabbits than I've got right here, even if you could sell them."

"Well, maybe you could teach me how to raise them. I'll start my own business!"

"Ah, the *meschuga kapitalist* [crazy capitalist] is at it again," he laughed. "I don't know if I should be a party to your crazy schemes. . . ."

Nonetheless, Mischa gave me all the tips and secrets I needed for raising rabbits. He was a good teacher and he didn't harangue me with his politics very often. In fact, I think it sort of amused him that his young neighbor was interested in starting such a non-kosher enterprise as the raising of rabbits in the middle of a major Jewish settlement.

I raised two kinds of rabbits: the white ones with red eyes, and the chinchilla type with gray salt-and-pepper fur. Since my father was a good carpenter, he helped me build the cages out of broken orange crates and chicken wire.

The raising of rabbits isn't a simple matter but, by trial and error and with invaluable advice from Mischa, I slowly became an expert. I figured out how to maintain high standards of hygienic living conditions, as well as how to cope with problems of infertility and of cannibalism by the mothers of their babies. Eventually, I had to come up with enough grass to feed almost seven hundred rabbits daily, which was particularly difficult in the dry season. Using some extra-legal initiative, I usually rounded the grass up from other plantations without permission!

As with any enterprise, the marketing of my product was very important. I had a few local customers, but not enough to make all my extra work worthwhile. By luck, however, I found the perfect market. It was the height of World War II and, though the Allies had started to have some success, we all knew that victory over Fascism was a long way off. Food rationing was a fact of life. We were allocated only a quarter pound of frozen, fatty meat from Argentina every month. The same was true with sugar: we were allocated only a small, shrapnel-like hunk.

In contrast, the soldiers in the British Eighth Army had everything. I used to watch them stop at the only big cafe in the village, called Bauchwitz, to buy all the booze they could drink and to get sorely lacking romance from willing waitresses. I knew all this because I had the patriotic duty of waiting outside for the moment when the military truck was left open and unattended by the boozed up soldiers and then grabbing weapons and other supplies for the Jewish underground, the Haganah. Although the Haganah was a secret organization and you never really knew who was a member, a few of the local members were assigned to marshal the forces of village children in stealing badly needed weapons.

By this time, there was a growing mistrust of the British because of their policy of controlling immigration so tightly. Besides, it was known that a substantial portion of the British administration in Palestine was pro-Arab. So the underground was preparing for the future. Of course, we kids didn't know all this: to us, heisting weapons and supplies was like a game! I never really felt that I was stealing since I wasn't taking the stuff for myself. When I stole a handgun it would disappear magically into the huge bra of our lady agent, Shoshke.

"If we stole a cannon," we joked,"would you have room for it, Shoshke?" She was not amused.

The Eighth Army also included a division of Poles from Sikorsky's Polish Army. They were nice fellows, but they were always ridiculed for having more officers than enlisted men. Some of them even spoke German, so it was easy for us to communicate.

One day, while parking Hyman, Dummkopf and the cart near Bauchwitz, I was approached by a half drunk, three-star Polish general.

"Hey, kid, what are you doing with those rabbits?"

"Oh, I'm trying to sell them but, as you know, they aren't kosher."

"Who cares!" he replied, "I will give you 2 pounds apiece for these. If you can get me fifty to a hundred butchered and dressed animals each week, I will pay you two and a half pounds per head. But be sure to leave the eyes in!"

I knew that I had hit the jackpot, especially since he would be paying me in British pounds. It would probably be worth more than I could make in a month peddling vegetables. I immediately thought of the seven hundred rabbits I had in cages at home, and began converting them into cash . . . quite a mercenary thought!

I did my duty to the Haganah by stealing a handgun, ammo, a helmet and some badges, and returned triumphantly home with my double success. Suddenly, I had become a purveyor of meat to the Polish division of the Eighth Army. I felt like a real man!

The next morning I awoke with mixed and confused emotions. I was excited about my deal with the Polish general, but I was still a child and loved my rabbits. I had my favorites, especially Squeaky. She was a fat mother rabbit who, rather than bite me, would lick my hands and caress them with her floppy ears. Although I knew I would get used to it, the idea of killing the rabbits was extremely distasteful to me. The rabbit suffered for just an instant, but I had grown up convinced that animals had souls and individuality, and killing my rabbits seemed like killing my friends. After all, I had been responsible for their lives from conception. I knew that killing a hundred at a time was really going to be hard. But I also knew how much we needed the money!

Uncle Karl's check for 100 pounds had finally arrived six months after Mom had written to him, but that money was quickly spent. Mom had given the check to Papa to buy materials to build our long-awaited house, a wooden frame structure with a corrugated tin sheet roof and a plywood interior. With his stubborn fetish for accuracy, Papa spent lots of time making sure that everything was square and level. I was more worried about getting the house built before the rains came! But well before the house was finished, Papa announced that all the money Uncle Karl had sent from America was gone. The house wasn't even half finished! A home with no roof was like having nothing at all, and we didn't have any money to finish the job.

However, as I have learned throughout my life, God is great and had mercy on my sick mother, for it was just then that my contact with the Polish general materialized.

Now, my father was very ambivalent about my rabbit enterprise. He was particularly reluctant about his own participation because he had adhered to a very strict vegetarian diet for forty-two years and found my rabbit enterprise morally questionable. Also, he had a very sincere love for all living creatures.

So, when Papa learned I would slaughter a hundred rabbits the next day, he was upset. "I really feel like opening the cages," he said, "and letting these rabbits of yours escape!" Fortunately, he didn't carry out the threat.

The next day was butchering day.

I killed my rabbits five at a time. Sometimes I would automatically give them a stroke of affection just before they received a heavy blow on the back of the head from my *nabutt,* a straight branch from a wild orange tree. After the blow they would give a violent jerk in the air. When they were dead, I cut their throats and the blood gushed out from their jugulars. The whole process didn't take even a minute and was, according to my mixed child-adult rationale, just about painless.

The next step was skinning them. This was done by cutting the skin loose around the legs and neck and peeling it back. I was able to accomplish this within a few seconds. Next, I stacked the skins in a pile; each was later salted and dried in the sun. The last step was to cut the guts out and flush the body cavity with water from a garden hose. I did not remove the eyes, which just kept looking at me, dead and helpless. I never did figure out why General Brodezky wanted the eyes left in. I suppose that must forever remain a Polish secret.

My Polish general was absolutely punctual. On the appointed morning at ten thirty-five, his jeep climbed the steep, sandy road to our orange plantation, pulling a covered trailer full of oblong ice blocks.

His appearance made me laugh. He was tall, very skinny and balding. The empty shoulders of his uniform made the three stars on his epaulets into dangling bells. But, he was the personification of order and bureaucracy. His driver and batman, Private Yanush, was one of the few enlisted Poles I ever met. The man was short and fat, and had a big nose with a red tip; the pants to his uniform were held up by some miracle under the bottom line of his impressive belly. Though he was almost always drunk, Private Yanush could still drive most of the time. He was very loyal and obedient to his noble superior, considering his services to the General a duty to God and to Poland.

As soon as the car arrived at our rusty farm gate, Yanush jumped out of the car, opened the other door and ceremoniously saluted General Brodezky as he walked through the gate. There was a grotesque aura about the General; swaggering through our arched gate, he acted as though he were passing through the Parisian Arc de Triomphe. Brodezky was all business as he went straight to the long wooden table where my one hundred butchered rabbits, individually wrapped, awaited purchase.

The General insisted that Yanush inspect each carcass and tag and number it with a felt pen. Yanush must have had a little more to drink than usual that morning and he had trouble inspecting the carcasses. He couldn't seem to count them accurately. One time he counted one hundred, then ninety-nine, then a hundred and one. Suddenly he let out a strange gasp.

"Look, that little Jew is selling us butchered cats!" he yelled.

The General hurried to Yanush as if a scorpion had bitten him. He grabbed the suspect carcass and turned to me.

"You little Jew bastard, you are trying to cheat us Polish people again and. . . ."

"What a stupid allegation!" The General towered over me, but I had a butcher knife in my hand. "The leg bones in a cat and a rabbit are completely different. It's common knowledge," I said, quoting Mischa's explanation to me a month earlier. "And, secondly, if you question my integrity, Mr. General, take your business somewhere else — preferably Nazi-occupied Warsaw."

The General, taken aback by my authoritative tone, retracted the accusations immediately and showered Yanush with Polish curses, the meaning of which I could only guess. He apologized in a most sincere way, paid me in cash with a handsome tip to clear his conscience, loaded his car and retreated, leaving me unrepentant for my outburst, still clutching my knife.

In retrospect, I knew that the poor Polish soldiers had lost their homeland and were strangers in a strange land and I was later ashamed for my lack of respect, but the Pole's anti-Semitic remark was just too much for me to take.

I stood at the gate a few minutes holding that incredible stack of crisp, green British pounds. It was unreal. Me, little Yehudale, earning such a sum of money.

"Wait 'til Mom sees this!" I thought.

I stormed into the shack with all my twelve-year-old chutzpah and walked straight to my mother's bedside. I gave her a loving kiss and pressed the 250 pounds in crisp English bank notes into her hands.

"Mom, you see, it was worth all the hard work. Now Papa can finish the house and you'll feel better soon."

Papa was sitting in his work clothes. My eyes met Papa's, and even today I cannot fully comprehend what went through his head. Was it sadness that the money came from the slaughter of the rabbits? Was it anger, feeling that his young son had outdone him? Or was it gratitude and pride for having a young son with so much ambition? After a few minutes of silence Mom handed the stack of bills to Papa.

"Pinja," she said, "Please go right now to Presman at the lumber yard and buy all you need."

The same evening, Papa returned home with all three of the village's horse-drawn carriages loaded with everything we needed to finish our home.

That night I had a hard time falling asleep after all the excitement of the day. When I finally did, I had a dream. Some of the lumber turned into half-rabbit, half-rat creatures that were climbing frantically on the frame of our house and destroying it. All of this was accompanied by frightening shrieking and sad music. One rabbit-rat looked exactly like my beloved Squeaky, whose offspring I had mercilessly butchered. I knew her by the black star on her white fur. A jury of a hundred rabbits sat in judgement, chanting "Murderer, murderer!" Finally, Squeaky got up close to my nose and started to chew on it. . . .

I let out a scream which woke even Papa. I was soaking with sweat.

"Yehudale, why did you scream?" Papa asked.

"I dreamt about the rabbits," was all I could say. The details, I felt, were too private.

V

The Rabbits and My Bar Mitzvah

✳

The construction of our house progressed by leaps and bounds. Papa hired Mr. Perlstein, a family friend and carpenter by profession, to help with the more difficult parts of the construction. Mr. Perlstein put aside all other work in order to finish the doors and windows for the house. Papa even ordered first class screens to keep out flies and mosquitos; he had always been irritated by my constant killing of these God-created creatures, even though I did it mainly to keep them from bothering Mom.

We worked up to sixteen hours a day in the hot summer sun to bring the house to completion. The main reason for our hard work was Mom's deteriorating condition. By now she grew tired so quickly that she could barely be out of bed for more than fifteen minutes at a time. I couldn't understand why she was so skinny all over while her belly was so big. Anyway, we hoped the new home would make her feel better.

I greatly admired my Papa's carpentry skills. He did a beautiful job on the house. On their Saturday visits our friends and neighbors would inspect it and give their approval.

Finally we started to cover the roof with corrugated tin sheets. Papa had bought the top grade because he wanted to be sure the roof over our heads was the best that money could buy. Stout-headed nails, imported from England, were to be driven into the roof to fasten and seal it. Papa decided to hammer the nails into the gullies of the panels instead of at the high point because he wanted to be sure that the nails would hold well in the wind. I suggested that we ask Mr. Perlstein for advice before going on with the roof, but Papa insisted that he knew what was right. We had done two-thirds of the roof that way when Mr. Perlstein came by to deliver the windows. Out of curiosity he climbed up onto the roof, only to see me nailing in all the wrong places.

"You stupid boy, stop nailing immediately!" he screamed at me, "You will ruin the whole roof and the house will leak all over forever. Wait until I tell your Papa. When he comes back he'll be furious!"

My eyes were so full of tears, I choked on my words and couldn't even stand up to Mr. Perlstein's fury. I lay on the roof hugging the hot tin, sure that it was ruined for good, and me with it. At that moment Papa returned from his break.

"Pinja," Mr. Perlstein said, still excited in his anger, "Your son, that no-good, cocky little shrimp, has damaged your roof. Look how he has put the nails!"

"Wait, Mr. Perlstein," Papa said, swallowing his pride, "I told him where to drive the nails. It was even against his judgment." We finished nailing the rest of the roof the right way.

We had lived in our new "palace" for two weeks when the rainy season started. Luckily, we had put Mom's bed under the part of the roof which was nailed in place correctly. Where I slept, I got soaked. The house leaked in at least twenty places and Mom put twenty different kinds of pots and pans all over the house to catch the water. Fortunately we had just built balatot floors, concrete covered with mosaic tiles, and so they were not damaged by the water. We had all the *mumchim* (specialists) of the trade come to inspect the damage and got plenty of advice. We tarred the roof and it melted in the sun; we cemented it and it cracked, and so on — but the part of the roof we had nailed on wrong always leaked, and whenever it rained we had to resort to Mom's stop-gap method for catching water. I still remember that from each pot came a special tone as it filled with drops, making heavenly music.

Thanks to the General, I was just loaded with money in those days. I bought myself a new pair of shoes, but most importantly, I got a new two-wheeled cart with rubber tires to substitute for the metal ones I had, so it was easier for Hyman and Dummkopf to pull. I had even managed to train Dummkopf to pull the wagon with Hyman in unison, an amazing feat considering the IQ of that donkey. You can imagine how I felt going through the village wearing my new shoes, in my new wagon pulled by two donkeys, with all the villagers looking out their windows!

One day I tied the donkeys and wagon right by the window of my favorite barber and entered to get my hair cut. Since I had made a reservation, I sat at the window chair, cockily swinging my legs to show off my new shoes.

"How is the great merchant today?" asked Ahron, the barber.

"Wonderful," I answered with a voice full of condescension for the simple barber.

"Well, do you want your usual cut?" Ahron asked, "Or would you prefer the new Yul Brynner style?" That year everybody's cinematic hero was Yul Brynner, the imaginary King of Siam, with his "elaborate" hair style. Ahron approached me with his hair clippers.

"I think I would make a great king," I said.

I was joking, but in Ahron's mind I had given my consent and before I could even open my mouth, he mowed a wide track through the center of my scalp. My blond locks lay like freshly cut grass on the floor. All the guys in the shop were laughing about "Tricky Ahron." I was fuming and a lot less puffed up.

I paid the barber for the haircut and walked out of the shop with a fabricated smile. I woke Dummkopf and Hyman and fled home as fast as I could. My blond hair was gone; I looked like a convict. The haircut hadn't made me the King of Siam or even the baron of my own village. I felt like Samson, whose strength was robbed by treacherous Delilah, but in my case it was even worse: a mere barber had fooled me.

"What is going to happen when everybody sees me looking so ugly?" I asked Hyman, for I needed someone to talk to in my moment of grief.

My biggest worry, however, was that — to my complete amazement — the head hidden under my typical round European haircut had distinct Mongolian features. In fact, the only thing that hinted at my Jewishness was my imposing nose. So there I was, Yehuda Gideon, the shaven and shorn giant, crying like a little baby on my way home from the cunning and mischevious barber. I was badly in need of motherly hugs and consolation.

Mom was shocked. I couldn't even begin to explain the chain of events but told her it was the work of dastardly Ahron, who would be punished someday by God and/or me. Mom kissed me on my almost bald head, but continued to stare.

"Yes, I know," I cried, "I don't look Jewish anymore; I look like a Mongol! It's terrible!" A river of tears choked me again.

"What has happened to our Yehudale?" said Papa when he walked in.

"That Ahron tricked him," Mom explained, "Now he looks like some Tartar!"

Papa sat down in his big chair, asked me to sit close to him and started to talk to me. I will not forget that father and son session if I live to be a hundred and twenty years old.

"Yehudale," he told me, "you are a very special kind of Jew, a descendant of a people called the Kazhars. They were Mongolian tribesmen who lived in the mountains and valleys between the Caspian and the Black Sea. They were excellent warriors, merchants and great horsemen. Their rule extended all the way to Moscow, Hungary and Turkey. They were exceedingly rough and did not believe in God — just the sword."

"However, one enlightened Kazhar ruler decided that his people should convert to Judaism. Now this was mainly out of political expediency because the Kazhars were sandwiched between the Christians in the South, the Moslems in the East, and the heathen in the North. Converting to Judaism helped them maintain their non-aligned, neutral status among warring factions. Their kingdom thrived for many years, but eventually the Kazhars were overrun, and small groups were scattered throughout Europe and Asia. All this was centuries ago, but that's why you have such different features. Your ancestors were Kazhars who settled in what is now Russia." He pointed to me and then to himself. "That's why we both look different than most people around here. You should be proud of it, even if they call you Genghis Khan!"

I gave a big hug and kiss to my bearish Papa and jumped up to look in the mirror. Yes, I was a Mongol, just as those wild horsemen in the movies! In my mind's eye, I galloped on a beautiful black horse, a long sword in my hand, brandishing it right in front of Ahron's barbershop. . . . For a week or two my "haircut" was the subject of considerable gossip in our little community of Ramatayim. But fortified by my Papa's personal history lesson and the knowledge that my blond tufts of hair had begun to grow again, I didn't really mind. Besides, all the attention seemed to help my business because everyone wanted to hear the story of the Kazhars!

Of course, the real controversy was not my looks but my non-kosher business enterprise. A constant and heated discussion of my rabbit selling circulated around our district of Sharon. It provided a spicy topic, viewed differently depending on each person's degree of religious orthodoxy.

The "moderate" adult groups felt that it was not proper to raise trefa (non-kosher) meat, speculating that with the same amount of effort I could have raised chickens or fish. They seemed to forget that chickens could not live on orange grove weeds and that fish need a pond.

The more liberal citizens of the "left block" felt that in a time of war, I had the right to produce food of any kind to feed the people. They even pointed out that in the concentration camps, people were forced to resort to cannibalism. The only problem they saw was that killing animals for profit had an undesirable influence on a child's character. They felt that my father, the vegetarian, should have led me in the right direction.

As I said before, Mischa, the Communist, was at first troubled by the blatant capitalism of my enterprise. But after some reflection, he felt that feeding the Polish troops who came to us via Russia to fight the common Fascist enemy was noble. He reasoned that even Stalin, his Communist god, would approve of my activities on tactical grounds.

To my peers I was the object of envy mixed with admiration. My pockets were always full of money. I felt the Polish tips were mine to keep, and as a result I got my first taste of "commercial friendship." I often treated my gruschless (penniless) buddies to such luxuries as chewing gum, ice cream, and their favorite snack, sunflower seeds, considered a real treat in the Middle East. Among my friends I also became known as a banker, because I would sometimes make "big loans" which were repaid with interest. I soon learned that for all of my wealth I was not necessarily liked, but in a poor kids' world I was at least seen as someone to respect.

The religious citizens, of course, were quite unhappy about my enterprise. Mostly they just shook their heads at me and saved their comments for my Papa, who really didn't care about what they thought, since he had little respect for those he considered "overly religious."

Rabbi Dravin, however, was not so closed-mouthed. He was extremely vocal on the subject of the rabbits! One of the few paid functionaries in Ramatayim, he received a salary from the Jewish National Council, the governing body of the Jewish settlements under the British Mandate. He was the official religious authority in our village, respected by many, hated by others, but feared by all. He was tall and extremely well dressed, usually wearing a shiny black silk coat and a big black hat. He had piercing black eyes, a long nose, and a full black beard trimmed to perfection.

One of the reasons he was so powerful was that in addition to his duties as rabbi, he was responsible for the issuance of the Teudath Kashrut, the kosher certificate which every food-related commercial establishment — from grocery store, to delivery service, to restaurant — needed to survive. To obtain a certificate, merchants had to pay a fee and also hire a mashgiach (supervisor) recommended by the rabbi to inspect their premises and supervise operations to make sure everything was handled in accordance with kosher dietary laws. God help anyone who needed the certificate and who fell out of the rabbi's or his supervisor's good graces!

When I started my non-kosher commercial rabbit-raising enterprise, the rabbi saw it as a direct threat to his kosher kingdom. He let everyone know he felt the enterprise was morally wrong. More than once our neighbors told us I was the subject of the rabbi's Sabbath morning drascha or sermon. He accused me of moral decadence and of contaminating the Holy Land and its people by producing non-kosher meat. In his religious fervor, he even alleged that this sinful practice just might further delay the arrival of the *maschiach,* the Messiah, for whom we had been praying for nearly two thousand years!

Actually, as is frequently the case when someone tries to make a major issue out of something relatively minor, the result of the rabbi's efforts had the effect of actually improving my business! Those who weren't inclined to buy my rabbits before, began to see me as the "underdog" in a fight with the powerful rabbi, and bought from me just to show support. Even those who wouldn't dream of buying my rabbits showed their support by extra purchases of vegetables. My business flourished! I did, however, make sure to stay far away from the rabbi to avoid any direct confrontations.

Summer ended and it was nearly the New Year and Yom Kippur, the Jewish high holidays. Riding Hyman home from school one day, I saw an elegant, shiny black car parked in front of our rusty farm gate. It glinted sharply in the bright sunshine and even made Hyman nervous. I was not impressionable, nor was I known for being shy. I was quite accustomed to visitors in cars. After all, I had a working relationship with a Polish general which (overlooking small details such as rank and age) I felt was based on mutual respect. Still, there was something special about this car; I couldn't wait to find out who was visiting.

I jumped off Hyman, tied him to the first tree I saw and even neglected to offer him a bucket of water. I ran to the door of our new home, caught my breath, slowed down, and entered like a mouse. There were three very important-looking guests sitting in a semicircle around Mom's bed. My father saw me come in and at once introduced me.

"Please pardon his sloppy appearance," said Papa apologetically, shaking his head at my untucked shirt and rumpled pants. "He's been out riding on Hyman, his donkey."

Of course Hyman had nothing to do with how I looked! I was always a mess. But I knew these must be really important visitors for Papa to make excuses.

"Yehudale," said Papa in a solemn, proud voice I had never heard him use before, "I want you to greet Professor Rabbi Zager, formerly chief rabbi of Prague, Czechoslovakia."

I shook his hand, looking up at this skinny, bearded man with white hair. He had a friendly smile! How different from the always serious and stern Rabbi Dravin. I could hardly believe he was a Rabbi.

"And this is the wife of Professor Dostrowsky, Yehudale," said Papa introducing me to an elegant, white-haired lady who gave me a looking-over worthy of General Brodezky.

Papa had told me many times of his adventures with Professor Dostrowsky during the pogroms of Odessa, but that hadn't meant much to me. What impressed me in those days was that he was the personal skin doctor of the kings of Egypt and Jordan and all their wives and children. Can you imagine the honor of touching and trying to cure all their skin ailments? Even being admitted into their harems! I was disappointed the professor himself hadn't come to visit.

The third guest was rather young. She was the daughter of Mrs. Dostrowsky and her name was Roni. She was dressed in a shiny British military uniform and was quite self-assured. She was one of the first women to enlist in the special Jewish Palestinian brigades to fight the Nazis. "It's her day off," explained Mrs. Dostrowsky. "We prevailed on her to drive us out here to visit your mother."

The formalities were over. Papa brought orange juice and tea to serve to our guests who were now seated close to Mom's bed. Suddenly Mom spoke to the rabbi faintly.

"I pray to God to live to see my son, Yehuda, at his bar mitzvah."

I was shocked. First, that she felt her days were numbered; second, that she wanted me to have a bar mitzvah. Although we had always been a very traditional household, we were never religious. The bar mitzvah is the religious celebration held when a boy reaches the age of thirteen, and officially becomes a man. It is much more important and solemn than ten birthdays put together, and the number and value of the gifts received are also greater in proportion.

"Now, Ella, this is nonsense," interjected my Papa. "Yehuda became a man at age nine, when he began selling fruits and vegetables to help support the family. We don't need a ceremony to confirm his *mitzvot* [good deeds]." Then Mama started to cry. It was a sad scene.

Suddenly, Mrs. Dostrowsky asked Papa to come out for a walk saying she wanted to see our beautiful orange grove.

"Yehudale," said the Rabbi at the same time, "Why don't you show me your rabbits? I hear you have quite an enterprise."

"You want to see my rabbits?" I asked incredulously. "Rabbi Dravin hates them! I know they aren't kosher, but they are beautiful."

"We know that all animals are created by God," said Rabbi Zager in a rather friendly, professorial tone. "Even those that are not kosher. So long as you only sell them to non-Jewish people, I don't consider that a sin."

I liked this rabbi instantly.

"But you know," I said once we were outside away from Mom, "Rabbi Dravin really does hate my rabbits. He always tells me to get rid of them. I am ready to bet he will really give me a hard time about them if I have a bar mitzvah."

"Well, let's not worry about that yet," he replied as we reached the rabbit hutches.

I proudly showed him my favorite rabbits and explained the details of my business with the Polish general. "One thing I know, Rabbi. These rabbits will like you better than the General."

"Why is that?" he asked.

"Because they know you won't eat them!"

The rabbi smiled and continued to observe them from a distance. He wouldn't pet any of the rabbits, which I couldn't understand because I felt their pelts were gorgeous. Perhaps he was afraid of their non-kosher contamination after all.

"Very nice work for a boy like you," was all the rabbi said, and we walked back to the house. Papa and Mrs. Dostrowsky were deep in conversation outside the front door. I saw Papa shrug his shoulders and nod his head, and Mrs. Dostrowsky gave him a big hug.

"Yehuda," Papa announced, as if from a high podium, when we were all back inside, "We have decided that in order to further your Jewish and universal education, and in accordance with the wishes of your mother, you'll have a bar mitzvah and Rabbi Zager will prepare you for it. I want you to know that it is a great honor to have a chief rabbi teach you."

Papa served more tea and Mrs. Dostrowsky stirred in a big teaspoon of Mom's orange concentrate jam, in the Russian style of tea drinking. She paid Mom a tremendous compliment by commenting that the jam was the best she had had in years. Mom's eyes lit up and she gave our visitor a jar of the jam to take home. Mom's smile was like that of an angel in heaven, and deep down I knew she might be there soon.

Papa made the financial arrangement with the rabbi, a flat fee to be paid after the successful completion of my bar mitzvah. Mrs. Dostrowsky gave Mom a hundred-pound note as an advance on my bar mitzvah gift. "Use it to buy everything you need for the big party to follow the celebration, Ella. I know you want everything to be perfect." I guess she must have known how hard-up we were!

Soon the visit was over, our guests got into the black sedan, Roni got the car in motion, and within a few seconds only a dust cloud over the sandy road remained of the auspicious visit.

"I'm afraid Rabbi Dravin won't let you have the bar mitzvah," Mom cried after they left, "And it's all the fault of your rabbits!"

"Ella, would you please stop?" Papa said in his deep, strong voice, "bar mitzvah or not, we have got to make a living and that's the way Yehudale helps support the family. Do you want me to be a beggar?"

Suddenly Mom started to laugh and waved the hundred pound note like a flag.

"Gidi," she called out, reverting back to my old name "You are sure lucky with these kinds of gifts. Now, you can buy some decent clothes and not look like a sloppy farmer."

"Don't worry about it," I said to Mom, giving her a big hug and speaking what was then, and still is, my favorite phrase whenever there is really something worth worrying about. "I've got connections, so don't you worry. You need to get well for my bar mitzvah. I'll take care of Rabbi Dravin. I am good friends with his daughter." (In fact, the girl had even touched some of the dried white rabbit pelts once, when I told her that the rich ladies of Jerusalem had their coats made of them. Of course I swore never to tell on her.)

Mom quieted down after these reassurances, and held out the money to Papa.

"Pinja, tomorrow, first thing, take this money to Rabbi Dravin and pay him his fee. Get a receipt so that we'll know that everything is arranged and final."

The next day Papa got on Dummkopf's back and rode straight to Rabbi Dravin's office, which was attached to the left of the synagogue and shaded by a large palm tree and a lopsided fig. Papa never got to talk to Rabbi Dravin, probably because of my rabbit business. But he did see the *shames*, the administrator and dues collector. Papa filled out some forms the shames gave him and then asked how much it would cost.

"This is a free service," the *shames* said, "However, large tips for the Rabbi and the shames are in order. The usual amount is fifty pounds for each and there is no receipt available."

Papa's blood pressure shot up. He was ready to walk out, but he stood there squeezing the hundred pounds, trying to control his anger. He remembered Mom's tears and caved in. Papa knew that the money would just disappear into the pockets of the rabbi and the shames and that the payment had nothing to do with the "free" ceremony. He handed over the money and slammed the door on his way out.

Of course, I was in school when all this happened so I didn't find out about it until several months later, which was very aggravating because, if I had known, I would have had nothing to do with the shames or that rabbi. Anyway, when Papa came home he kept quiet. "Everything is fine," he said.

During those days, Mom's physical condition fluctuated. Some days she insisted on cooking a big pot of orange peels, which she would use for her famous jam, but within an hour she would be exhausted and we would have to call the doctor. When the fluids in her abdomen made her too uncomfortable, we took her to the Beilinson hospital where she would stay for two days of treatment. The frequency of these visits gradually increased and I began to wonder how long her health could last.

Meanwhile, I was studying diligently with Rabbi Zager, who came to our home once a week. He was a wonderful teacher and I immediately overcame my misgivings about participation in a religious ceremony.

"We are Zionists, you know," I told him on his first visit, "not religious. We hardly ever go to synagogue and Papa never goes. I don't think he likes religion."

"Well, Yehuda, it's not enough to be a Zionist. To be a true Jew, you must know and cherish the Jewish tradition. Rebuilding the physical state after two thousand years of destruction is only meaningful if you understand the culture and tradition that gives shape to the building of the Jewish homeland. Your father knows this. I'm sure that is one of the reasons he agreed to the bar mitzvah.

"These next few weeks will give you the opportunity to learn about our people through our prayers and music. Did you know that some of the world's first musical notes are part of the Jewish heritage?"

Before I knew it I was engrossed in learning and looked forward with anticipation to every weekly session with Rabbi Zager.

The final session before my bar mitzvah took longer than usual. There was a full moon, but it was still too dark for the old rabbi to walk to the village alone. He was glad when I decided to accompany him. After we had walked about a third of the way, on a little hill overlooking our green valley, Rabbi Zager stopped.

"Yehuda, I want you to listen to this chant," he said.

He sang the *Kol Nidre* for me and for the moon and the stars and the growing field, possibly for the world itself. His voice, though old and tired, had a depth and beauty that I had never heard before. The *Kol Nidre* is a prayer from the time of the Inquisition in Spain. It has to do with the forced conversion made by many Jews to avoid execution and exile. "All my vows are null and void," the prayer says, renouncing the promises to Catholicism and reaffirming Judaism.

"Yehuda," he said when he finished, "In these few lines and this simple melody you can feel all the sadness, greatness and eternity of our people. You should be proud of your heritage.

"The Jews who created the prayer of *Kol Nidre* in Spain, the *marranos*, risked their lives to preserve our heritage. This heritage is the basis of great civilizations.

"Yehuda, I want you to be a proud Jew in *Eretz Israel*."

I was never the same after that evening on the moonlit hill. The Rabbi captured my heart and mind.

Preparations for the bar mitzvah went smoothly. The packing house, our former residence, was transformed into a dining hall. The wooden packing tables were covered with white paper fastened with thumbtacks. For chairs we turned 250 orange crates upside down. Lots of neighbors appeared at my Mom's bedside, even my Aunt Chana from Haifa came for the week to help out. It was the only way to get ready for the huge crowd arriving Friday afternoon for the Saturday morning ceremony.

Papa may not have been an expert farmer, but he was still appreciated by his numerous friends who remembered his exploits in Russia as a young man, his dedication to Zionism and socialism in Vienna, and his efforts on behalf of the Zionist movement in Palestine. He was not a politician, but he had close relations with many of them. And many were planning to attend my bar mitzvah.

Papa rented all six rooms in the only hotel in the village. There he placed Professor Dostrowsky, Ben-Zvi, who was later to become the second president of Israel, and the rest of the V.I.P. guests. Other guests found places to stay in the homes of local friends and relatives. Food preparation for two hundred and fifty was no small problem in time of war; in 1943 everything was still being rationed. But my brother Dov, the big-shot sergeant-major, had pull in the community; in this way he was able to secure extra rations, so that even the food problem was solved. Papa also had friends who helped even though he didn't ask them. Everybody in the village knew me as the little big mouth who had his hands in everything, so even some of my friends pitched in.

Finally, the great Sabbath arrived. I was dressed in my new suit, bought with rabbit money. Papa was decked out in one of his sharp suits salvaged from Vienna. It was the first time I had seen him in a suit since we arrived in Palestine. Dov was dressed in his meticulously pressed uniform with his shiny badges and ribbons. His shoes were shining like mirrors and he wore his five-gallon felt hat. He was very impressive.

Even my mother was dressed in a white dress with a few blue ribbons. The day before, the doctor prescribed medication to pep her up for the next day. And that morning she was feeling better. She had waited for this day, the day her son would become a man, for thirteen years.

The ceremony in the synagogue was planned for ten o'clock. I harnessed Hyman and Dummkopf to my wagon and filled it with pillows so that Mom would be comfortable on the ride. Normally it is forbidden to work with animals on the Sabbath except in life-threatening cases, but I was sure Rabbi Dravin would agree that this situation was life-threatening, since walking would have killed my mother.

They helped Mom walk from her bed to the donkey wagon, tall Dov on her right and Papa on her left. I was too small, so I kept the donkeys in check. When they arrived at the wagon and tried to help Mom into it, she suddenly collapsed. It was no use.

"I can't make it," she cried, "Take me back to bed!" I choked back tears. It broke my heart to see her. Papa looked like he was about to cry too. Only Dov was composed. He quickly carried Mom back to the house to rest.

The crowd in and around the synagogue was far greater than the population of the village of Ramatayim. We approached the synagogue, Papa on my right, Dov and Rabbi Zager on my left. The guests formed a double line of honor leading to the shrine. Through the double door, I was able to see the center of the synagogue festively draped. Above it were the two tablets with the Ten Commandments inscribed on them.

Out of nowhere appeared the *shames*. He approached us.

"Mr. Sorokin, could you please step into Rabbi Dravin's office immediately?"

We knew something was wrong, but what could we do? Papa and I met the rabbi in his study; the room was loaded with books and he sat behind a big table in traditional black garb and wide-brimmed sable hat. His stern, penetrating stare scared me; to me, he looked like an agent of Satan.

"Well, Mr. Sorokin," he said, "I'm sorry to approach you at the last minute before the ceremony, but the *shames* in his hurry forgot to have you sign an agreement that your son will stop raising his disgusting, non-kosher rabbits. I will take your word of honor since it is the Sabbath day and we cannot write. You are known to be an honorable man."

Papa turned white. First Mom's collapse and now this. He nearly fainted and had to sit down.

"Can I get you a glass of water?" the *shames* offered. Papa leapt up with all his strength and grabbed my hand.

"Rabbi," said Papa forcefully, "If you would have put this condition a month, a week, or even a day ago I could have answered 'yes' or 'no'. But to force this agreement on me five minutes before the start of the ceremony is wrong in the eyes of God and all decent men. This is nothing but blackmail. To agree to something just because two hundred and fifty people from all over the country are here, including national leaders of the Jewish community, is wrong. You must change your mind."

The Rabbi with a face of stone said just one word, "No."

We left the Rabbi's office, and my Papa explained to the crowd that there would be no bar mitzvah. Everyone was stunned. Some shouted, calling it a disgrace, but most just walked quietly down the main street of Ramatayim behind Papa to the converted packing house dining room which was all prepared for the celebration.

Papa and I went into the house to tell Mom that there would be no bar mitzvah after all. She turned pale when she heard about Rabbi Dravin's actions.

"This Rabbi thinks he can play God, Pinja. I am horrified." I heard her say to Papa in a low intense voice. I don't think I had ever seen her so angry.

"Well," he replied holding her close, "we must make the best of it. We have a whole houseful of people here to help us celebrate, and after all, we do have something to celebrate. Yehuda did complete his studies with Rabbi Zager. What difference does it make if we don't have a formal ceremony. It's the preparation for the ceremony that is meaningful."

With that, Papa picked Mother up and carried her to the head table in the converted packing house, which was by now filled with our guests.

Professor Dostrowsky was seated opposite Papa and Mama at the VIP table. He was small and stocky and completely bald, and very distinguished; his wife Sonja, a very elegant lady. Professor Dostrowsky's experiences had taught him to be soft spoken but resourceful. The room was buzzing with conversation as everyone talked about the rabbi's refusal to proceed with the ceremony. When everyone was seated, Professor Dostrowsky stood up and the room froze in silence.

"Dear friends," he said, "We came from all over the country to celebrate the bar mitzvah of our dear Yehudale and to honor his parents. This despicable act by Rabbi Dravin is an attempt to destroy this day for all of us. I am sure that in the eyes of almighty God, Yehuda made more mitzvot than any of us adults. He has sustained his parents and, in particular, his ailing mother. I have never met a young man like him. We wish, in the presence of all of his relatives and friends, that he grow up to be a man our nation can be proud of."

The whole crowd raised their glasses and with the traditional blessing of *leychayim* (to life) the wine was consecrated.

I got up from the table after Professor Dostrowsky's speech. I needed a moment alone and some invisible force pulled me to the rabbits. I opened one cage and hugged the first rabbit I saw. He laid his floppy ears on my chin.

"I don't care, bar mitzvah or not," I told him, "I love you, my rabbits. You understand me better than any of them."

With that, I returned to the packing house filled with guests. The tables were filled with fruits, cakes, hot *falafel, pita, humus* and steaming Turkish coffee. There was an atmosphere of *simcha,* festivity, despite the disappointment of the morning's events at the synagogue. Outside, the younger guests had started to dance the *horah,* a passionate, fast dance done in a circle. Inside, those who did not dance joined in singing pioneer songs followed by nostalgic songs from their former homelands.

When the last guests departed the sky was pitch black, studded with millions of stars and a half moon.

Later that night I had a new version of the old nightmare. This time, in the center of the synagogue, I saw the rabbi dressed in black. He was running around in a panic, chasing the rabbit-rat creatures. They were gnawing on the rafters of the building with frightening shrieks. I was watching this scene from the window, panicking myself. Then I lifted a bucket and tossed its liquid contents through the window. The synagogue was instantly transformed into a flaming inferno and the rabbi disappeared in the smoke.

At that moment I let out a terrible scream. I woke up in my bed sweaty, shivering and surrounded by my whole family.

Papa had the final word, which I still remember many years later. "Well, Yehudale, none of us will ever forget those rabbits and your bar mitzvah."

VI

The Donkeys

*

*I*n the Middle East when I was growing up, the donkey was a very important part of daily life. Of course we children used to race against each other on our donkeys, but the donkey was mainly a means of transportation.

Everyone used donkeys to carry fruit and vegetables to market. Bedouin women would load their donkeys with bales of fresh-cut grass or firewood collected in the fields and they usually walked in front of the donkeys, dressed in their long black traditional costume. On their heads they balanced their *jarra* (terra-cotta containers) full of water since they of course had no running water in their tents. Even today, donkeys play a major role in Bedouin life. The Bedouins travel in small caravans. The men ride up front on the biggest donkeys, followed by their wives, on foot, who lead a less impressive donkey loaded with an enormous pile of household goods. From the donkey's saddle a rope runs to the first camel's neck, then to the next camel and so on, so that the whole group paces in unison through the sand dunes — a sight far more facinating than a row of cars stuck in traffic!

I used to ride my donkey Hyman to school every day, mainly because I was born with flat feet, which in my youth were always painful and forced me to wear special shoes. Since we lived about five kilometers from school, Hyman was a blessing. Besides, my social status was enhanced by being able to bestow a special favor on the kids I liked by having Hyman carry their school bags home.

I used to tie Hyman up near the school fence, leaving him a bucket of water and some weeds to eat. He would wait patiently for me while I was busy getting smarter in class. Every now and then he would bray, a distinctive baritone, in the middle of Mr. Moses Schlanger's lesson on the greatness of some Biblical hero or prophet. Mr. Schlanger would glare at me as though it were my fault that Hyman chose that particular moment to bray.

As I've said, my other donkey was Dummkopf, so named because her scant mental capacity. She was much smaller than Hyman, had reddish hair and was quite attractive for a donkey. Though not as strong as Hyman, she was a good worker and reasonably obedient, although she frequently imitated Hymans deeds and stubborn suggestions. Like many redheads, she was quite amorous, at times showing too much affection and irritating him. She would lick him and nibble his neck, while would feign displeasure and kick her in the shins.

Believe it or not, I think I was probably the first farmer in Palestine to plow with two donkeys in tandem. The main agricultural product in our region was citrus. Endless citrus groves, called pardessim, extended beyond the horizon in all directions. In the late fall, the trees looked as though they were studded with round gold nuggets. In the spring, their snow-white flowers produced a sweet, seductive smell that on balmy nights made you feel as if you were in Shangri-La. Of course, the citrus trees needed lots of care: watering, fertilizing, spraying and plowing to loosen the soil.

When I was growing up, the plowing was usually done by a medium-sized horse, guided between rows of trees. The problem was that horses were generally too tall for the job and large portions of the land could not be plowed. One day when I was about fourteen, Papa and I were watching the hired *balegula* (horse and buggy driver) and his horse do an unsatisfactory job.

"Papa," I said, "Hyman is half the size of a horse. If we used him we could plow much closer to the trees."

"Why not, Yehudale," said Papa, laughing, "Maybe you could get the job done even faster by using Dummkopf. Hyman would probably kick and run to try to get away from her advances!"

It irritated me that he didn't take me seriously, and this strengthened my resolve to prove I was right. As soon as my Papa and the balegula left, I took the plow and changed the setting to medium depth to compensate for the fact that donkeys have less strength than horses. I hitched the donkeys to the plow, putting Dummkopf on the inside because she was smaller, and Hyman on the outside where the major pulling action was required.

Once or twice Dummkopf tried to provoke Hyman by kicking him with her delicate rear legs, directing her blows at a place that would hurt. But Hyman behaved like a gentleman and ignored her. I, nevertheless, let her know that I didn't approve of those shenanigans on the job! After a few light lashes with an orange branch, she got the message and didn't try anything more.

So off and away we went, the first tandem donkey plow operation.

After an hour of trial and error, we got it down pat. The *balegula's* plowing job was terminated, I got the additional duties of plowing our *pardess* twice a year and we saved a great deal of money.

Now and then, Dummkopf or Hyman would get hurt during a plowing session. Once a sharp branch punctured Dummkopf's side and blood spurted everywhere. For a moment she went berserk, but was quieted by the petting of Hyman's twenty-inch long ears. I had learned, from one of the first-aid sessions I had attended at school, that in the absence of more conventional medication, you should use urine to flush out a wound. I tried this and also applied a pressure bandage made with one of my socks. And indeed, the wound healed in a few days. It was my first experience as a doctor and I was immensely proud.

The plowing of the *pardess* took a couple of weeks because the donkeys and I were unable to endure more than two working-hour sessions a day, one before school and one after school. On the very last day of the plowing season when we were close to the pardess gate, Hyman suddenly jumped off his front feet in terrible pain. He had stepped on a nail. He jumped around frantically, trying to dislodge the nail. I was terrified. I could see the nail sticking out of his foot, but had no idea what to do. I unhitched him as fast as I could in spite of all the thrashing around he was doing, grabbed an orange branch and tried to hit the nail with it.

Finally, it worked and the nail fell to the ground. Hyman's foot was bleeding profusely and he was limping badly. My father somehow blamed me for Hyman's accident.

"How negligent to have let him step on a nail," he said.

"Don't you think we should call the doctor?" I said. I had never heard of veterinarians before.

"You are right about that," Papa said, "Get on Dummkopf immediately and ride to Doctor Ellenberger who lives on the hill in Kfar Mallal. He is the only veterinarian around. Tell him what happened and ask him to come as fast as he can."

Off I went. Dummkopf, it seemed, did not understand the urgency of our mission. She simply would not move fast enough, even though I urged her on with my riding crop and more than a few curses! When we finally arrived I discovered that Dr. Ellenberger had a telephone and we could have called him!

Well, Doc Ellenberger was a very impressive *Yeke* (most doctors in Palestine at that time were *Yekes*).

"Ja, ja," he said, on hearing my story, "This is urgent. You might lose the donkey."

"Can you save him?" Now I was really worried.

"I think so. After all, what did I spend all those years in the university for!" he replied, "But I'll need a good assistant. Can you stand the sight of blood?"

"Of course!" I answered proudly, "I have butchered over five hundred rabbits, cutting their throats and dressing them!" I embellished a little, I have to admit, only stopping short of saying I loved the sight of blood.

Well, I'm not sure whether he was convinced, but he said I could be his assistant. He sent me on ahead; he was going to get ready and come back with his horse and buggy. "Much faster than your miserable little donkey," he told me. I was so excited about being his assistant that I ignored the insult to Dummkopf.

Doctor Ellenberger arrived with his shiny horse and carriage. In the coach were many drawers filled with his equipment and medicines. There was even an icebox for the supplies that needed to be kept cool. He stepped down from the wagon and went immediately to Hyman, who was standing there, strangely quiet and woozy. My Papa told the doctor what had happened, and that he had wrapped the foot and leg with a white sock to prevent it from becoming contaminated with dirt. In the Russian tradition, Papa had also given Hyman a bottle of vodka to help kill the pain. No wonder Hyman was swaying so!

Doc Ellenberger ordered me to lift the injured leg and to remove the sock. He then put the foot into a pail of soapy water. Hyman stood quietly, probably because he was completely drunk. After washing the injured area, the doctor swabbed it with concentrated iodine, a solution that must have hurt a lot, but didn't even make Hyman moan. Dummkopf, who was watching the proceedings from a short distance, let out a bray, seemingly a cry of compassion for her beloved companion.

A compress bandage full of iodine ointment was wrapped on the foot, but the main event was still to come. The doctor pulled a small vial from his icebox.

"Anti-tetanus serum!" he announced.

He filled a syringe, then placed a sponge soaked in alcohol in my hand and told me to wash off an area of Hyman's hindquarters.

"Every veterinarian's assistant must know how to give shots," he said, startling me by putting the syringe in my hand.

Well, I was scared, but even more cocky. I was determined to do it. I got the needle into Hyman's leg, injected the serum and was thrown promptly into the sand from the force of a swift donkey kick. Still, I felt victorious. I had given my first injection! Later, when the story became known in the village, I was nicknamed "Little Doc." I was very proud.

The doctor ordered a two-week work furlough for Hyman, which meant that I had to ride Dummkopf to school and I didn't like the idea at all.

As was the custom, the vet was invited to tea, which my mother still made despite her poor health. Papa, Doctor Ellenberger and I sat at the table, complimenting my mother on her cake and sipping tea. As usual, my father and I drank the tea in the Russian style with plenty of lemon and thick homemade jam. The doctor was amazed at our tea-drinking habits. A typical Yeke, he couldn't understand anyone drinking tea differently from the German style.

I remember he spoke highly of my doctoring skills to my mother. He didn't even mention Hyman's kick and my quick descent into the sand. When he left, my mother called me to her bedside with a glowing face.

"My son, the doctor," she said, "You are all I have to hope and dream for. Promise me you'll become a doctor, Gidi. I know I won't live long enough to see it." I burst into tears, knowing she was right, she would not live to see it. It would take me thirteen more years.

The story of my doctoring spread, my reported treatment of poor Hyman becoming more and more elaborate every day. Of course, I gave updates on the patient's progress daily at recess. One of my best friends, a devout animal lover, even visited Hyman on our farm, bringing him a watermelon and a get-well card. Although I thought this was a bit extreme, Hyman appeared grateful. He first split the melon into many pieces and ate the center, the sweetest part. He then devoured the entire watermelon, the rind, the paper wrapper and the gift card. Watermelon was splashed all over his face. I was very pleased at the appreciation he showed for the gift.

Hyman did improve daily. I was treating him every day, which mostly meant soaking his hoof in a warm disinfecting fluid, a secret concoction of the doctor's. And every day I reported his progress to Doctor Ellenberger, waiting for his scientific approval.

"You do a wonderful job," he would tell me, "A real vet couldn't have done better."

It made me feel so important.

Even Dummkopf behaved extraordinarily well during this trying time. Once, she even pulled out a big *rigile* plant, with its round, juicy leaves, and instead of eating it herself, she carried it between her teeth directly to Hyman and dropped it for him to eat. Hyman looked at her with affectionate eyes and she stroked his leg with her ears. When Hyman let out a loving bray, I knew real romance was on the way. Shortly thereafter, Dummkopf began to mysteriously gain weight, and Hyman became very protective, trying to bear as much of the load as possible, as is customary for a Papa-to-be.

Months passed and Dummkopf's pregnancy became very obvious. The kids at school were quite interested, as none of my classmates had ever seen the birth of a donkey.

Well, the day when Dummkopf's contractions began and some lemony fluid mixed with blood began oozing from her privates, I knew it was her time. I was nervous. I was supposed to go to school, but instead I jumped on Hyman and rode as fast as I could to Doctor Ellenberger's. I had forgotten that he had a telephone. Still, Hyman galloped so fast I'll bet he outdid an ambulance.

But all that effort was to no avail. Mrs. Ellenberger greeted me with the news that the doctor was in bed. The horse of Moishe, the *balegula*, had given him such a bad kick that he couldn't walk for two weeks! I was devastated. What was I going to do? Ellenberger was the only vet; the next closest lived in Petach Tikva, which was very far away. I begged Mrs. Ellenberger to let me talk to the doctor. She disappeared into the house for a few minutes. When she reappeared she invited me into the bedroom. It was such a great honor!

Doctor Ellenberger was lying on his big brass bed with his injured leg wrapped in an ice compress. His face was fat, but pale. He groaned a little as he spoke to me. I explained Dummkopf's situation, the bloody fluid and the contractions, which were about fifteen minutes apart.

"Well, my junior assistant," the doctor addressed me in very serious tones, "You'll have to do it on your own. But don't worry, most of the time that *chamor katan* (donkey foal) will arrive into the world of its own accord. The only thing you have to be sure about is that the head lies between the baby's stretching legs as they emerge. If, God forbid, one leg isn't there, you are in trouble.

"Then you'll have to put oil on your hands, push the head back in and then pull the missing leg out. If you can do that everything will be fine. Be sure to tie her up well and have your Papa help you lift her tail so you can do the job right. If you need advice, call me on the phone. You will miss school today by the time this is all done. But those lessons can wait. This will be a very important experience. God bless you in this."

I was surprised by this last remark. I never knew Doctor Ellenberger was religious. No one had ever seen him in synagogue.

I was back home in a flash. Hyman must have grown wings. Papa was standing around, pacing nervously around Dummkopf, helplessly looking at the protruding mouth and single hoof emerging from the donkey's privates.

"I don't know what is going on with Dummkopf. It looks as though the baby is stuck!" he said. Then he looked around wildly, "Where is the doctor?"

"I am here," I said proudly, but not without a little terror in my heart, "And the doctor has told me just what to do." I explained to him what had happened.

I gritted my teeth and plunged into the job, ordering Papa to move Dummkopf to a corner and hold her tail. My friend Lulach, a six foot giant, happened by just in time to help stabilize the donkey in the right position. I washed my hands diligently, as well as Dummkopf's privates.

I doused my hands with oil and tried to push back the foal's head.

"You are making it worse, Yehuda!" Papa screamed.

"Patience!" I growled, too busy for his outburst. I was having quite a time with the head; it wouldn't budge. I was too weak to move it at all during the frequent contractions and could just barely budge it between them. Then I remembered Lulach.

I ordered him to push my hand, which in turn was pushing the foal's head. But my hand was so slippery with oil that when he pressed it, it shot forward with the head into Dummkopf's insides. It was warm and slippery and I reached deeper and deeper, feeling for the second hoof. When I found it, it was a moment better than any I could remember. I tugged at the leg, bringing the head back out with it. We all paused.

Suddenly, Dummkopf let out a loud bray. With one last huge contraction the whole foal came out. A true miracle of nature. Papa was stunned and Lulach was strutting around with pride. It was true that I could not have done it without him. I took an old towel and scrubbed the mouth and nose of the newborn. Then I cut the umbilical cord and tied it in a knot and cleaned it with iodine. The baby began to breathe regularly and then, stumbling like a drunk, he tried to get on his feet. It took him ten minutes.

I was so pleased!

Dummkopf began to have more contractions and Papa decided she must be having twins. I put my hand back inside and checked before I said, with a know-it-all air using the phrase I had only just learned from Dr. Ellenberger, "It's just the afterbirth!"

As the little donkey went for her first meal at her mother's teats, we considered what to name her.

"Let's call her *Mazal*," Papa said, using the Hebrew word for good fortune, "Because she was so lucky you knew what to do, Yehudale. Without you, she wouldn't have been born."

I liked the name my father chose, and especially his explanation.

We cleaned everything up and off I went to school on Hyman. If it was hard for him to leave his first foal, he didn't complain. Maybe it was his way of thanking me.

After about a week's maternity leave, during which Hyman performed all duties, Dummkopf came back to work. Mazal had grown strong. She had a beautiful, deep, Bordeaux-red coat. I loved to pet her. She was still nursing from her mother, who had plenty of milk.

It was the eve of Passover and I had lots of orders for Valencia oranges. My father filled the little wagon to the brim while I was at school and I hurried home, eager to sell the oranges so we would have money for our Passover meal. The wagon was just too heavy for Hyman to pull alone, so I had to hitch up Dummkopf and let little Mazal follow freely along. Away we went.

Everything seemed okay. Hyman and Dummkopf were pulling the wagon and I had decided to walk in order to reduce the weight they had to pull. Mazal was following behind her mother, a little to one side.

But suddenly the local bus appeared, loaded with people hurrying home to prepare for the holiday. Simon, the driver, was in his lane when Mazal darted in front of the bus. Dummkopf saw Mazal headed for the bus and lost her wits. With unbelievable strength, she pulled Hyman and the wagon with her, breaking free of my reins. I watched in horror as the bus smashed into the wagon, scattering oranges everywhere.

When I finally caught up, I saw Mazal, lying in agony with both front legs broken and pinned between the bus and the wagon. I knew she couldn't be saved, except from her misery. I had to act quickly. I pulled out my Swiss Army knife and slit poor Mazal's throat. The baby donkey barely winced, she was in so much pain that she was unconscious already.

I felt sick. Blood was everywhere. Smashed and splattered oranges covered the road and the front of the bus. Somehow, I pulled myself together and apologized to everybody; to the passengers, who were pretty shaken up, and to Simon, the driver. It was such an awful sight. I loaded up the wagon with what I could save of the scattered oranges and returned home with Mazal's little body. I had to tell Papa.

"You could have been killed," he gasped, hugging me. "Mazal was certainly given the wrong name," he said later.

Well, life had to go on. I knew that young donkey meat was a great delicacy to some, and very expensive. So I decided, without telling my vegetarian father, that I would drag Mazal's body to the rabbit butchering area and dress it. Although I had butchered a lot of rabbits, this time the butchering was especially heartbreaking because Mazal was the first-born of the two donkeys I had grown up with. But it was still wartime and it would have been a sin to let anything go to waste.

I pulled the skin, cut the legs and head, cleaned out the innards and divided the carcass into eight pieces. Donkeys, like rabbits, are not kosher and therefore not to be eaten, according to people like Rabbi Dravin and his book of law. However, in my book, it was okay as long as you were not Orthodox. I put the cut-up carcass in an orange crate, and headed toward the house of my all-important brother.

Dov was now married. Eva, his wife, was a very beautiful woman who, though somewhat overweight, was utterly adorable and had a heavenly operatic voice. Their home was simple, but clean and nice, full of mementos of my brother's military escapades. Eva's feelings toward me varied a great deal. On one hand, she admired my commercial talent and my veterinary inclination, because she was a nurse. But on the other hand, she thought I was a little bastard who always had his way.

That evening Dov wasn't home, so she was by herself when I knocked. When she opened the door, I dropped the crate at her feet.

"Happy Passover," I greeted her.

"Yehudale," she said, "What brings you here?"

"I just wanted to show you how much you and 'the General' mean to me," I told her, "I was very lucky today. As you know I have become the veterinary assistant to Doctor Ellenberger. Today, I assisted him with the birth of twin calves." I went on to exaggerate my veterinary skill greatly, which wasn't hard to do since the whole story was pure fabrication!

"One was perfectly normal, the other had three eyes and something wrong with his mouth. The farmer didn't want him, so he gave him to me for my services, along with the biggest watermelon I have ever seen. I gave the watermelon to Mama and Papa. Papa didn't want the meat, of course, so I thought I'd bring it to you and Dov."

"This is wonderful!" she gasped. She lifted the cloth covering the crate and said, "But where are the head and feet? I would have liked to have had them too."

"No, no," I said, "They were deformed. Trust me, they couldn't be saved." I galloped home on Hyman, laughing all the way at the trick I had just played on Eva.

VII

My Mother's Funeral

＊

The most beautiful animal in our village was Blacky, the horse. I used to pass by him every day on Hyman. Each day I admired his beauty anew. He used to stand at the center of our village, hitched to Moishe the balegula's work wagon. The horse's pitch-black shiny coat, gentle intelligent head and elegant legs made him stand out from the ordinary horses waiting for work to begin. It was as if he were lowering himself from some aristocratic position to be a simple draft animal. To me, he was a horse above all horses.

Blacky always led our village parades. In the May Day parade, he and his wagon were draped in the red flags of the workers' movement and the blue and white Star of David flag. Blacky carried the local big shots, sometimes even leaders of the Jewish National Council, when they visited. And don't be fooled that Blacky wasn't aware of its importance.

Other important jobs were also reserved exclusively for Blacky. He was the horse who pulled the funeral wagon for our village. What a sad honor. Sometimes, as I was passing by, the thought would occur to me that we might soon be needing Blacky's services. I knew that the time was drawing near.

Although a number of years had gone by since my mother's experience with the Nazis, her hands never really got better. They always oozed and caused her constant pain. Her weakened heart went from bad to worse and the emergency visits to the hospital became more and more frequent. My Papa was devastated that he, who was so strong and vital, could do nothing but stand by and watch his wife's candle of life flicker dimmer and dimmer.

Mom lost weight until she was just skin and bones. Her belly grew bigger and bigger with fluids that had to be drained ever more frequently. Finally, during one of the doctor's visits, I saw him and my Papa walking away from the house together. They spoke quietly and seriously. The next morning we took my Mom to the hospital and Papa told me she would need to stay a long time. But it was not so long after all.

I went to see her every day after school. On the fourth day, she was so weak she could hardly speak. She seemed incoherent. I bent down to kiss her and somehow I knew that was the last time I would ever see her alive.

"Gidi, be a doctor," she said. These were the last words she said to me.

We stayed late that night as she slipped into a coma. Finally, exhausted, we went home. In the morning Dov appeared to tell us that the hospital had called him at the police station. Mom was dead. We all began to cry. I went to Mom's empty bed, touched it and closed my eyes, trying to pray. I directed my thoughts and feelings toward heaven and wondered if Mom was there now with Minka, Mrs. Billig, or maybe even Mazal.

Papa was devastated. Without Mom, even with all his physical strength, he was helpless. Dov seemed to take Mom's death stoically, like a soldier should, I suppose.

Because of the heat, it is the custom in the Middle East to bury the dead the day of their death. It is also the custom according to Jewish law. In every Jewish village there were a number of respected elders, religious men called *chevre kadishe,* who prepared the dead and assisted in the burial. Usually the rabbi would give a eulogy at the grave site. But Papa specifically asked that Rabbi Draven not participate in our hour of grief.

We immediately notified Moishe, the *balegula,* to bring Blacky and his black flat bed wagon for the funeral procession.

Where we lived, there were very few funerals because, in those times, the population was very young. So a funeral was not only an occasion of sadness and respect, it was an opportunity to dress up in the best clothing we had to wear. Funerals were also social occasions, with the number and status of the participants adding to the solemnity of the event.

Hundreds of people came to Mom's funeral. I really don't know how the word spread so fast. But that day in the late afternoon, when a sad red sun started its slow descent into the sea, an enormous procession followed the *balegula* and Blacky as they pulled the black wooden coffin carrying my mother. We stopped at the green, rusty double gate to our farm, as if to let Mom's soul say its final good-bye to the land she cherished so much but enjoyed for so little time.

Suddenly, Papa's friend Mendel Singer, a well-known journalist, opened a blue and white flag with the Star of David and draped it over the black pall covering Mom's coffin. The crowd froze.

"This flag was saved from the *Blau-weis,* blue and white movement in Vienna, where our dear friend Ella gave her youth for the cause of the land of Israel. It is customary to drape coffins of our leaders and soldiers only. But Ella was wounded by the Nazis and still fought the battle of our people to the bitter end. During her last few months in Vienna she supported our people, comforted them, found ways to help the condemned in Dachau, supported orphans and aided the sick. She joins the mothers of our people as one of the heroines of our national movement."

I was stunned by his words. I had been completely ignorant of what my mother had done during the time I was in the orphanage. She never told me of her activities.

Dov and seven other policemen walked alongside the wagon slowly. Blacky held his head high as the wagon moved through the narrow sandy road in the direction of the cemetery.

It was May and the orange groves were in full bloom, as if a million flowers were dedicated to Mom. The heavenly perfume helped to lessen our grief. Blacky made the final turn into the cemetery and the coffin was brought into a special room by the *chevre kadishe,* who washed the body and draped it in white linen. You see, Jews believe that in our final resting place both rich and poor are the same. In the *tachrichim* (Jewish burial garb), there are no pockets for carrying worldly possessions into the grave.

The crowd surrounded the grave site. My brother and his policemen friends carried the coffin to the grave. There the coffin was opened and my Mom's draped body was placed in the bare grave. The sight was unforgettable.

The cantor started to recite the *El maley rachamim,* the merciful God prayer. I was crying harder than before. I couldn't see God's mercy for my mother. She had suffered so much only to die at the age of forty-three. I could see no justice. While the cantor continued the prayer, close friends were given the honor of shoveling soil to cover my mother's body, and soon she disappeared forever.

Papa was composed, but stunned by his loss. Dov stood at Mom's grave with the empty expression of a soldier. Only I was crying. The cantor came and said, "Yehuda Gideon, son of Pinchas and Ella, please say the Kaddish prayer in memory of your departed mother." As if by magic my tears ceased and I said the prayer in a loud clear voice, sanctifying God in Heaven, and praying for everlasting peace for my mother. At the end, I added my own words in an even stronger voice.

"And God please avenge the blood of my mother and all the innocent brothers and sisters now in the hands of the Nazis."

The crowd was stunned by my emotional and unorthodox addition, and started to disperse slowly, placing flowers and wreaths on the grave.

Finally just Papa and I remained. I knew this was the final farewell. I still had in my hand the only two roses from the bush that grew in front of our house. I fell on the grave, crying, and attached my two roses to the wooden grave sign.

Moishe offered to take us home. We climbed on the wagon and he let me take the reins. I commanded Blacky to get moving and the fresh air of the evening stroked my skin, with the stars and the moon out in all their glory. The wagon and its gentle sway in the sand made me feel as if I were airborne, flying by the moon and stars toward my Mom who was now in Heaven, telling her, "Don't worry, I'll be worthy of your memory. I'll fulfill all of your wishes."

Blacky's loud neigh brought me back to earth and reality. At our farm gate we all descended, thanking Moishe for all he had done. I stroked Blacky's head with affection while he looked at me with sad eyes.

Within a month a permanent grave stone was erected on my mother's grave. Engraved on it are my small hands holding the two roses, and the inscription, "To Mother." I still miss her.

VIII

Spies, Sniffing Dogs, and Fish

*

O ur neighbor Mischa was not the only communist in my life. My Papa's adopted sister Chana and her husband were also ardent communists. Chana's story was extraordinary. She had been an abandoned baby, wrapped in rags and placed on the step of the synagogue where my grandfather Dov found her. Imagine what would have happened to her in the rough Russian winter if my grandpa had not happened by! Grandpa named her "Chana," which means "merciful," and throughout her life she lived up to that name.

Shortly after he rescued Chana, grandfather died of pneumonia which he caught after crossing the village at night in a terrible snowstorm. Grandmother and little Chana were supported by my uncle Syoma, Papa's older brother and a general of the Cossacks. My Papa and Chana parted ways during the Russian Revolution: Papa was active in the Zionist Socialist movement, and Chana was dedicated to Communism. They eventually lost track of each other completely after my father escaped from Russia and ended up in Vienna.

When we arrived in Palestine, Papa found Chana, by sheer coincidence, at the workers' May Day Parade. Papa had just finished marching when he looked up and saw the flag of the PKP (the Palestine Communist Party) and a small group of marchers gathered to one side. There at the front of the group was a small, skinny woman with big glasses and a leathery face, a cigarette hanging out of her mouth. She was gesturing and talking excitedly, her wild, wavy hair blowing in the hot wind.

Papa immediately recognized her.

"Chana, can it be you?" he shouted to her in Russian, a language he rarely ever used in Israel.

"Pinja?" She ran to him and gave him a big Russian-style embrace, ignoring the fact that just moments before they had walked in the same parade, but under very different political banners.

Chana lived in the city of Haifa, in an apartment on top of a roof, with her husband and three children. They ran a dry-cleaning business on Herzl Street, and to save money did the actual cleaning in their roof-top quarters. Their apartment was always a mess. In fact, my fastidious Papa would never eat there because the place, especially the kitchen, was so unkempt. But Chana had a heart of gold. She worked at least fifteen hours a day, seven days a week. Most of the money went just to care for her three kids and the two orphans she raised in addition to her own children. The rest she spent on helping others, or donated to the Communist Party.

After my Mom died, Chana stepped in to try and replace her. She was always inviting me to Haifa for the weekend. She even introduced me to my first real girlfriend!

Aunt Chana's son Fila was in the Naval Scouts, a nautical equivalent to the Boy Scouts; he was crazy about boats and fishing. Fila was several years older than I, and I really wanted to be friends with him and have him take me fishing.

"Mom, he's too young!" he would exclaim whenever Chana suggested a joint outing. "He might fall overboard in the ocean. I can't take him with me. Maybe some other time."

"Be patient, Yehudale," she'd comfort me. "One day you'll be old enough to join the Naval Scouts on your own! In the meantime, you can help me eat the fish Fila brought me from his last trip, and dream about the time you will be able to bring home fish of your own. There will be lots of company here to entertain you this afternoon anyway. A whole group is coming over to discuss the government's attitude toward Arabs. I know you will be interested in the conversation." In short order she turned my irritation at being too young to go out with the Naval Scouts into pride at being considered old enough to join in important political discussions.

Chana was still a faithful communist. In fact, she was one of the leaders of the Communist Party in Palestine, much to Papa's disgust. I can still hear them arguing in our little one-room house. . . .

"Pinja," she would say. "I can't understand how an intelligent man like you, a man of justice and integrity, can continue to be supportive of a Jewish state. This land belonged to the Arabs. We need to live in peace among them. There is no need for a separate state. There is no reason to take their land!"

"A separate state does not preclude peaceful co-existence!" my Papa would respond with exasperation. "The trouble with you communists is that you are unrealistic. You think no one has a need for a state. Well, that may be true in philosophy, but not in the real world. The Jews need a Jewish state in order to survive! That's that. Even in Russia, where your precious communists are in power, the government created Birabijan for the Jews, recognizing their need for a state of their own! Of course, that experiment is doomed to failure because the Jews in Birabijan have no historical roots there as we do in Palestine. Even you came here, Chana. Would you have come if it weren't for those roots, the history of our people for over two thousand years? And don't give Yehudale any of your crazy ideas!"

The argument was always the same and neither Papa nor Chana could convince each other, but that didn't stop them from trying. I have to admit, I also thought my Aunt Chana's politics were a bit strange, especially since she worked so hard to earn money, which she then gave away to the Communist Party. As far as I could see, the party never did anything much for her except fill up her shop and apartment with people who wanted to talk politics!

Of course, politics was always a topic of conversation in Palestine. and there were always so many points of view! These subjects remained rather remote from me, however, until the summer before I went to high school. That was the summer I was initiated into the Haganah.

The British had been in Palestine since the end of World War I, ruling it under a mandate from the League of Nations. Early in the mandate, the Government of England promised that any Jew who wanted to immigrate to Palestine would be permitted to do so. Unfortunately, the reality of Middle Eastern politics led the British to cut back on that promise as they sought to maintain control in the face of growing Arab discontent and increasing Jewish pressure for a national homeland as promised in the Balfour Declaration.

Of course, the Jewish settlers had never relied exclusively on the British for protection in Palestine. When we arrived in 1938, there were three Jewish underground defense organizations in operation, all illegal: the Haganah, the biggest and most moderate; the Etzl, an extreme, terrorist oriented organization; and the Stern Gang, a splinter group of the Etzl, which was even more extremist, believing that any means for creating a Jewish state in Palestine was acceptable.

My brother Dov was in the Haganah. Mikve-Israel, the agricultural school where Papa had sent him to study, also served as a recruiting ground for new members of that organization, and Dov had joined very soon after he arrived in Palestine. Rather than going into agriculture following graduation, Dov joined the Jewish Settlements Police Force (the Gafirim) at the suggestion of some of the leaders of the Haganah. The British had created the Gafirim in order to give the growing Jewish settlements some additional protection from Arab marauders. That way, the Palestine Police Force, which was made up of Jewish, Arab and British officers, could avoid having to get involved in messy inter-community conflicts.

Very quickly, the Gafirim ended up serving as a British-paid cover for instructors of the Haganah, which was an all volunteer organization. The arrangement was very handy. Anything threatening to the Haganah which became known to the Gafirim was promptly passed on to the appropriate Haganah members. As the Gafirim also worked closely with the Palestinian Police, they were able to gather lots of information important for the defense of Jewish settlements.

One day shortly after I arrived from Vienna, when I was complaining about the fact that Dov never came to visit us, my Papa took me aside and told me to listen. Dov, he said, was in the Haganah.

"Yehudale, your brother is important in the underground. A commander. He works very hard in our defense. He can't come here just to visit when there is so much work to do. Now, you must never reveal what I have told you. It could jeopardize his life. I just wanted you to understand why he can't be as close a brother as you may wish."

"I swear I'll never tell," I replied, deeply impressed by the importance of my brother's responsibilities.

The summer before I went to high school, Dov himself finally let me in on his secret during one of his infrequent visits to the family. I still remember the scene. He arrived in uniform driving his motor scooter, which was the envy of most young men his age living in the area. But this time, instead of sitting down with Papa as he usually did, he said, "Yehudale, come with me for a walk. I have something I want to discuss with you."

I was surprised at the serious tone in his voice. When we reached the orange grove, he got right to the point.

"You know I am in the Haganah, don't you, Yehudale? I'm sure Papa must have told you."

I was afraid to answer, not knowing whether I or Papa would get in trouble.

"Don't worry," he laughed, seeing my confusion. "Papa told me that he had told you! Now I think you are old enough to join with us in some very important jobs, not piddly stealing of guns from drunk soldiers like you used to do when you were a kid!" I swelled with pride at his trust.

"We are badly in need of a 'slick,' a place to hide weapons used for training recruits. It's too dangerous to carry them back and forth to the training grounds."

"What do you want me to do?" I asked excitedly.

"I will bring you three big milk cans to bury, and later I will bring you weapons to store in them. You will have to do everything in the middle of the night, when nobody will see you. You aren't to tell Papa where you bury the cans. Only you, me and one other person will know. Don't tell Papa anything. This is very important!"

"I promise I won't tell him, I won't tell anybody!"

"Okay, but first you must take the oath of the Haganah. In a few days someone will contact you."

A week later I was standing at the soda fountain in the center of the village when a man I didn't know approached me. He beckoned me toward a corner of the shop. "Be at the end of Borochov Street under the big eucalyptus tree at 10:00 Friday night. Someone will meet you there. Be sure not to tell anyone about it. No one."

On Friday I arrived for my appointment ten minutes early. It was pitch dark and a cold autumn wind was blowing. There was nobody to be seen. I was shivering, and not just from the cold.

Finally, I felt a tap on my shoulder. I jumped! "Bo [come]!" someone I couldn't quite see commanded me. We walked silently for about one kilometer to a remote packing house in another *pardess*. There were about eight young recruits and two instructors waiting.

For about two hours we sat on the floor listening to a lecture about the founding of the Haganah in Russia, and the history of its expansion in Eretz Israel, where it grew out of the *Hashomer,* the defense organization for the original Jewish settlements in the Galilee.

After the lecture, as the candles lighting the room flickered eerily, we all stood in a circle and responded one by one to the leaders' questions.

"Yehuda Gideon Sorokin, are you willing to join with us in the fight to defend our people?"

"Yes," I responded.

"Are you willing to pledge allegiance to the Haganah and follow the orders of your leaders?"

"Yes, I am."

"Are you prepared to die, if necessary, for our cause?"

"Yes."

"Then put your hand on the *Tanach* [the Old Testament] and swear allegiance to the Jewish people and the Haganah."

The questions were repeated and answered by each recruit around the circle. In all my life I do not remember a more solemn occasion.

Two days later I stole out of the house while Papa slept. Dov's friend, Azriel, met me at the edge of the *pardess*. A truck stopped near the fence and unloaded three big milk cans which we promptly carried into the orange grove. They were big, but not too heavy, as they were empty.

We worked for several hours to dig holes big enough to hold the milk cans and so that we could cover them with at least five inches of dirt. "We want to make sure none of the dogs trained to sniff out explosives and weapons will find this cache, Yehudale," explained Azriel. " Be sure to cover the loose dirt with weeds that will root easily. We can't have any signs that would reveal any digging. And be sure to go home the long way around, on the road. Never come here by a direct route from your house. The trained dogs will find the trail if you do!"

The next day, Dov personally brought a big knapsack containing thirty guns of all different types: American, German, Russian, and Italian pistols. There was an assortment of ammunition and explosives as well.

"Yehudale, you'll have to grease every one of these guns to protect them from the moisture in the ground. The milk cans have a good seal, but we can't take any chances. We have so few weapons!"

It was messy work, and difficult to do in the dark with only a flashlight, but I was thrilled to be trusted with the job.

Soon Dov began to come with great regularity. He not only brought weapons to hide, he would sometimes take them away to use on night training missions. I was surprised to learn that some of the training was taking place in our own *pardess* and in the eucalyptus grove just above it, without Papa knowing about it since he went to sleep early.

Mysteriously, however, the Palestinian Police Force began to patrol our street as never before, directing bright spotlights into the yards and the orange groves. "Something is going on," my Papa said. "They aren't doing this just for fun." And sure enough, about two weeks later three Palestinian Police Force jeeps pulled up in front of our house. A contingent of officers swarmed into the house without knocking. Two of the men were leading big German shepherds: the dogs were sniffing everything like crazy. I watched with anxiety as they passed through the yard on their way to the orange grove.

The officers were very stern. "Mr. Sorokin," they addressed my father. "We have information that some illegal activities are taking place in this area, perhaps on your land. There have been reports of lights shining in the packing houses around here at night when no one would be packing oranges. And mysterious lights have been spotted in the orange and eucalyptus groves. Tell us what you know about this," they demanded.

"Why nothing. Nothing at all. I go to sleep early at night. I haven't seen anything," replied my father with absolute honesty.

"And what about your son who always seems to have his nose in everything? What does he know?"

"Yehudale? Why, he's just a boy. What would he know about your mysterious lights at night?"

"I haven't seen anything," I replied for myself. "I have to get up early to sell my vegetables. Then I go to school. I go to bed at the same time my papa goes."

By now the sniffing dogs were very close to the spot where the guns were buried. Fortunately, they stayed on our side of the fence! I had hidden the milk cans just over the edge of our property on the other side of the fence.

The officers left empty-handed. Papa looked at me with raised eyebrows. "So, you've been seeing a lot of Dov lately. That doesn't have anything to do with this mysterious visit of the Palestine Police, does it?"

"I hope not, Papa," I replied honestly, not wanting to lie or betray my secret activities with Dov. I went to bed that night wondering who had been spying on us and knew enough to tell the police.

Dov came the next day. "We'll have to leave this 'slick' alone for awhile and move the training efforts elsewhere. There's a spy someplace. It's too dangerous."

"Does that mean I won't have any more missions?" I asked with disappointment.

"So you like excitement, eh?" laughed Dov. "Well, you did a pretty good job. I think you're ready for some additional training. Go to Haifa to Aunt Chana for a few weeks before school starts. I will tell Fila to teach you how to help with beach maneuvers when we bring in refugees from the ships that make it past the British blockade."

"Fila? I thought he just went fishing all the time! It used to make me mad that he would never take me along."

"Well, now you know. His supposed love of fishing is just a ruse. He even buys the fish in the market and keeps them on the boat just for show. He really fishes for Jewish refugees!"

"Does Aunt Chana know?" I asked incredulously.

"Of course not!" he answered emphatically. "You can never tell whose side these communists are on! They worship Stalin and take orders from him! We know they spy on us whenever they can."

"Aunt Chana a spy? I will never believe that," I said.

"I don't think so, either," said Dov. "But you never know. . . ."

With that, he jumped on his motorcycle and disappeared in a storm of dust, leaving me to ponder the role of spies, sniffing dogs and fish in the struggle for a Jewish homeland.

IX

Chickens, Eggs and High School

*

*I*t was 1944, and World War II was moving into its final phase. The daily newspapers, and especially the newsreels, helped feed our sense of euphoria. Victory over Hitler's evil empire! We had not yet begun to understand just how evil.

I was fourteen, and it was still a relatively carefree time in my life. Interspersed between the newsreels were thrilling movies like Casablanca. I saw it three times, hoping a little bit of Humphrey Bogart would rub off on me. I practiced these long, sad romantic looks on my girlfriends whenever I could.

Papa now acted as mother and father to me. He also tried to do the housework, but he wasn't much good at it. I still remember the big box where he threw all the socks with holes in the toes. The pile just grew and grew; neither of us had any idea how to fix them, but my Papa couldn't bring himself to throw them out. Maybe he was expecting a second wife to mend them. Lot's of women were interested in him, but he never showed interest in remarrying. "I married Ella, that's it. No more." And the pile of socks kept growing.

Papa had always planned to send me to high school at the Hertzlia Gymnasium in Tel Aviv, the best high school in the country. In his usual, impractical way, he never gave a thought to the high tuition. Anyhow, one day, dressed in our best — I wore pants I had ironed myself with an off-center crease — we set off for my enrollment. Not one to miss an opportunity, I carried with me a small suitcase full of eggs carefully cushioned in newspaper. Rationing was still in effect, so I knew there would be plenty of black market sales opportunities in the city and we could get a much better price than in our village. In fact, I already had big sales schemes planned for the coming years when I would be attending high school. My little vegetable cart business at home would be curtailed by the time required for commuting to school, so I planned to sell eggs and chickens to my teachers and new friends in the city.

We rode the bus to Tel Aviv, then walked from the bus station to save the fare, arriving just in time for our appointment with the principal of the school. Mr. Bugrashow looked old and stern, even mean. Papa and I felt very humble in his presence. In his office hung pictures of the school dating back to the day of its founding. It was the first Hebrew high school in the world. There were pictures of former students too, some of them now important leaders of the country. The ideal of Eretz Israel and Jewish pride and culture were pervasive themes in the pictures. I was instantly drawn to the school and wanted to be a part of it.

Mr. Bugrashow interviewed me. I was nervous and didn't come across as well as I wanted. Then the matter of the two-hundred pound deposit came up, to be paid immediately with the application for admission. Papa, of course, was stunned; he had no idea the fee would be so high.

Unlike Papa, however, I was ready. I put the suitcase on Mr. Bugrashow's desk and opened it. Two hundred eggs were neatly lined up. I then reached into my pockets and pulled out a pile of bills, all jumbled up. They were my tips from the Polish general. I had been saving for years, just to be ready in case of need for a good cause. And what better cause than my own high school tuition?

Mr. Bugrashow was astounded, both by the pile of crumpled money, easily more than two hundred pounds, and by the sight of the two hundred almost-impossible-to-get-in-Tel-Aviv eggs. When he heard the story of how I had saved all the money and my plans to sell the eggs he said, "Well, you are certainly enterprising. Exactly the type of student we would like to have here! By the way, do you think you could spare some of your eggs?"

I knew I was in.

"Of course, Mr. Bugrashow. For you, a special price!" I put thirty of the brown eggs on his desk and he paid me.

"Have your son here on Monday," he said to my father. ("With more eggs," I thought.) "I will take care of all the formalities of admission." Those eggs not only helped to get me admitted, they saved us a lot of bureaucratic steps.

I spent four years at the Hertzlia Gymnasium and each day carried one or two suitcases full of eggs and butchered chickens. Many of the chickens came from our own farm, but a number of them came from our neighbor, Mr. Hyman, my donkey's namesake, who was delighted to have a daily marketing operation for those of his chickens that needed to be butchered immediately (before they died and couldn't be sold legally!). The price I paid him to acquire his nearly dead chickens for my salvage operation was modest, so I always had a nice profit margin on my sales to city customers. They were always willing to pay a premium for "chickens and eggs fresh from the farm."

Butchering the chickens wasn't nearly as distasteful as killing the rabbits had been, but the cleaning and plucking operation took some time. I had a long bus ride to Tel Aviv and had to get to school on time. It was a struggle until I learned from my neighbor, Mischa — the one who had gotten me started with the rabbits — that by dipping the butchered chickens in hot water, the feathers would come out easily and quickly. I didn't like his Communist politics, but he sure knew a lot of good tricks.

I usually arrived at school only one or two minutes before the starting bell, and I always left my precious suitcases with Saadia, the school's shames (maintenance man). He and his wife lived in a little house connected to the school building. There he would keep my chickens and eggs until the noon break, when a number of teachers would descend from their classrooms to buy them. I was in seventh heaven. Yehuda, the great entrepreneur, with his own teachers as customers!

My supply never exceeded the demand. I could have charged just about anything for those chickens and eggs, but I considered myself ethical and charged only enough to make a decent profit. Of course, I may have also considered that these same customers would be grading my school performance and that a little restraint (and from time to time a special break on price) might do me well.

I had very little time to study. I did most of my studying during the bus ride between the village and Tel Aviv, and a little at night by the light of a kerosene lamp.

Once I was very late to school because the bus broke down. Despite the extra time, I had not done my homework as I preferred to chat with the other stranded passengers. When I finally got to class, Mrs. Dvora, my biology teacher, asked me a question I couldn't even begin to answer. It was not the first time I'd found myself in such a sorry state of affairs, and this time she was angry.

"You come late. You are not prepared!" she scolded, "You're the champion of excuses. Well, you are about to get a D in this class. I'll bet you can not even dissect one of your own chickens and name all the parts!"

I knew when a cue was being handed to me.

"Oh yes I can!"

I ran to Saadia's house, grabbed a chicken and returned to begin my dissection and "lecture."

After a ten minute dissertation on the anatomy of the chicken I concluded, "The best is for last. You all thought this was a chicken. Actually it was a rooster." I triumphantly held up its testicles. "These are the ones that make it possible for him to take care of twelve females!"

The boys all laughed and the girls turned very red. Mrs. Dvora was not amused, but she got the rooster for her dinner and I got an "A" in the class anyway.

✳ ✳ ✳

By 1947, my third year in high school, things were not so carefree. The world had learned the full horror of the Nazi atrocities. Our innocent belief in the goodness of the United States was shattered by the knowledge that Roosevelt had, perhaps deliberately, avoided actions which could have saved thousands or millions of Jews. Thousands of Jewish refugees were desperately trying to enter Palestine, only to be turned away or interned in camps again, this time by the British.

Despite the danger of arrest, my friends and I, along with others in the Haganah, including my cousin Fila, would frequently go to the waterfront near Tel Aviv at night to help unload and lead to safety the tired and sick refugees — those who were lucky enough to be on a ship that made it past the British blockade. The refugees came by the hundreds. I will never forget the haggard, frightened faces of the men and women we carried with their shabby suitcases. Despite the terrors of their journey, their eyes shone with the knowledge that they were now free and safe.

Safe? Perhaps not. By 1948, the dream of a peaceful existence between the Jews and Arabs in Palestine was still held by only a very few. Those of us in the Haganah (most of my classmates were members) were now training to fight for our homeland. The British had become the enemy, clinging to their Middle Eastern power base. Despite the post-World War II global ground swell for an independent Jewish state, they were enacting ever more repressive laws limiting immigration and the rights of Jewish settlers.

Seeking to divide and conquer, they actually fomented enmity between Arabs and Jews. Finally, with the adoption of the United Nations resolution calling for the end of the British mandate and the establishment of independent Jewish and Arab states in Palestine, it became clear that war was imminent. Our graduation was moved up almost two months so we could join the army or the reserves and prepare for the coming fight.

I will always remember that ceremony. The whole school was seated in the inner courtyard, with the graduating class up in front. No guests or relatives were invited. Life was very difficult then, as everyone was preparing for war, and besides, there would have been no room for them in the small courtyard. We were all very somber and serious as Mr. Bugrashow stood before us to speak. He began by reading from the Tanach about Gideon and his warriors. I felt as if he were speaking directly to me and swelled with naive pride, eager for battle.

"I will be brief this morning, for it is with mixed emotions that I perform this ceremony which will send you out into the world. You came here as children. You leave as young adults. I have grown fond of you all and worry about your future, the future of us all. . . .

"Your years of study here were designed to prepare you for a life much different from the one you will now have to face. You are leaving us at a crucial moment in the history of our people. There will be unimaginable hardships for all of us as we try to create a new independent nation of Israel. I can only hope that the knowledge and love of your Jewish heritage, which we tried to instill in each of you, will serve you well. May it inspire you to fight, to defend your nation, and may it support you when the price for an independent Israel may seem too high. May God keep you safe. And remember the words of Herzl, the father of our country: '*Im-Tirzu Ein Zu Agada*. If you really want it, Israel is not a fable, but a reality.'"

✳ ✳ ✳

We left the courtyard three abreast, marching to a song of hope and leaving our childhood behind.

X

The Mule That Saved Me

✳

I was never so scared in my life as when I landed at the bottom of that trench, covered with blood. It wasn't even my own blood, but that of a mule.

"What happened to you?" cried Beni, my buddy, whom I had left groaning in pain just a few minutes before, when I went for help and medicine for his wounded shoulder. He thought I was worse off than he was; I certainly looked it. But it was just the blood of a dying mule caught in the crossfire.

✻ ✻ ✻

The year was 1948. It was winter and cold, with strong winds blowing through the cypresses and orange trees which surrounded the Arab village of Kfar Saba. This was the place of my first battle experience. Immediately after the end of the British Mandate, seven Arab armies had invaded Palestine from all sides, trying to annihilate the newborn Jewish state. Because my brother was in the army, and my father too old to fight or to manage the farm on his own, I was assigned to a reserve unit that helped guard the border between the Jewish and Arab territories: by day I worked the farm with Papa, by night I did guard duty with my unit. Finally, however, the situation was so desperate that even my unit was called to the front. I was part of the last of the reserves to go.

We were a rag-tag unit consisting of poorly trained citizens of various ages and walks of life. I was the youngest, as most of our troops were in their fifties. They called me a kid and, because of my age and relative speed, assigned me the role of runner between the various defense positions. The job was dangerous and I was frequently exposed to enemy fire.

Kfar Saba was just a cluster of mud huts, but the thick, reddish mud bricks were picturesque in comparison with the cement blocks in the Jewish houses of my own village. Kfar Saba was in shambles. Its inhabitants had gone into exile at the advice of the Mufti Al Husseini, leader of the Palestinian Arabs, who told them they should leave until the Jews were "pushed into the sea," at which time they would be able to return safely. "By the grace of God . . . it won't be long," he told them. Only abandoned dogs and cats, a few chickens and donkeys, and a big, brown mule remained. We called the mule "Poor Ahmed," I don't know why. The few animals left were wandering aimlessly in the deserted alleys of the village, here and there finding food and bits of grass. I'm sure they wondered what was going on, why people were killing each other, and what had happened to peace.

I could barely understand what was happening myself. I was certain that the Arab villagers had been very foolish to leave, and even more foolish to think that we would be pushed into the sea and that they would be able to return and take over our houses and property. After all, we had grown up in relative peace and harmony. It was unthinkable that we would have harmed them, unthinkable to be in a war and unthinkable that they would triumph. But here I was, in the battle of Kfar Saba which everyone said we couldn't lose, for if we did the Arab Legion would invade the heartland of the Sharon Valley within hours and finish us all. I knew I was fighting not only for my own life, but for that of the Jewish homeland.

In the Jewish villages only the very old and the very young remained. The rest of the men and women were at the front, facing odds of one thousand to one and a tremendous disparity in the quality and quantity of weaponry. I had been given a one hundred-year old rifle, manufactured at the time of Queen Victoria and probably heisted from some museum. Bullets had to be loaded one at a time.

My buddy Beni and I were locked in battle now against a sole Arab Legionnaire hidden in the village across an open field of two hundred yards. He had a modern machine gun, a Bren, at the time the ultimate in semi-automatic weaponry. Every now and then I could see his face across the field, and his sleek British-style uniform capped with the traditional red kafia (scarf). I had only to lift my head slightly out of the trench and he would send a spray of bullets. In return, I would shoot a single bullet, carefully aimed, but useless just the same because the sight on my gun was poorly calibrated. Our duel of unequals had lasted for hours, with no winner in sight.

Beni and I were weary, not to mention hungry and thirsty, from the tension and length of the fight. Food and water could only be brought in under cover of night, as the main road to the front was completely exposed to enemy fire. The next defense position, behind us, was only reachable across an almost open field.

Beni spied a cluster of oranges in the tree next to our trench and decided to try to grab the fruit. Without warning he jumped out of the trench, climbed the tree and plucked three oranges. He jumped from the tree directly into the trench, but caught a bullet in the shoulder as he leaped.

Expensive oranges! He was bleeding profusely. I pulled out my first-aid kit, not knowing what to do. I put a pressure bandage on as best I could. Although I really wanted to cuss him for his stupidity, I comforted him and gave him half a bottle of wine, hoping that would ease the pain a little.

Then I started to panic. The field telephone had stopped working and I had only five bullets left from my daily ration. With Beni out of commission, I was essentially alone, with very little training and no commander. Beni was getting paler all the time. The next defense line was too far for my cry for help to be heard, and besides, I was afraid my enemy would discover how hopeless and helpless I was.

Perhaps there really are a few heroes in battle, but I was just plain scared. I was pushed against a wall. I had to do something!

Then I saw Poor Ahmed, grazing near the trench, searching in vain for something edible. If he were just a little closer, maybe I could use him as a shield while I made a run for help! "The oranges," I thought, "Maybe he'll come for the oranges!" I tore one open so the smell would attract his attention and started making animal-like noises to call him over. Cautiously, I pushed a pile of the yellow fruit out a short distance from the trench, hoping the legionnaire wasn't paying too much attention.

Slowly, Ahmed wandered over, attracted by my vocalizations or the fruit, or just by luck. When he finally got close enough to smell the fruit, he moved more quickly, stopping at exactly the right spot to feast and help shield me. I jumped out of the trench, pushed by all the adrenaline I could muster as I ran the short, but exposed, distance to the next defense line.

Although it was less than a hundred meters, it felt like a kilometer. I dashed like an Olympic competitor; I was running for my life. As I reached the last two yards, the legionnaire unleashed his fire and hundreds of bullets zoomed around me. Miraculously, I reached the next defense position safely.

Quickly I told an older soldier, a medic, my story about Beni, but he was too old to try and run back to the trench with me. He gave me some better pressure bandages, a shot of penicillin, and some instant medical training on how to give injections to humans — it's different than with donkeys.

"I'll notify command," he said, "and try and get you some help."

"God knows from where," I thought. But his words were somehow reassuring.

I carefully crept to the edge of the covered area, waiting for my chance to return to the trench and to Beni. Poor Ahmed was still at the same strategic location, innocently munching on Beni's oranges. Suddenly, a terrible noise erupted from our command post and, across enemy lines, a fire broke out in a pile of hay. Because this was around the time that the Israeli "secret weapon," the Davidka, was making its first appearance, I feared I might be getting my first introduction to its use. Later I would discover that the legionnaire's weapon was just a rudimentary mortar, making a lot of noise and requiring a great deal of prayer to reach it's aim. At that moment, though, it seemed a fearful and powerful weapon. The noise, the explosion and the fire were terrible, and I was sure it must have scared the legionnaire. I hoped it had distracted him.

I remember I offered up a brief prayer. Though I can't recall the words, I am certain it wasn't one of Rabbi Dravin's meaningless religious conventions. I was scared and this prayer was really from the heart! Finally, I felt some courage building. The distance was short. Focusing on Ahmed, I dashed out from safety. For the first few seconds, everything was okay, but as soon as I reached Ahmed, a hail of bullets fell on us. Aimed at me, the majority pierced Poor Ahmed. Only one grazed the helmet I was wearing. I was covered with the mule's blood as I dove into the trench.

Beni was only half conscious. "What happened to you?" he exclaimed in horror.

While I applied the new bandage to his wound, I told him the story and then gave him the penicillin shot. Not very well, evidently, as Beni claimed that the injection hurt more than the injury! Soon he quieted down and drifted in and out of sleep. He was in less pain now that the new bandages were in place.

I took a break from my guard duty, still clutching the antique rifle of questionable combat value. A few yards from me lay Ahmed, dead, with his head turned in my direction and his eyes fixed on me, as if accusing me of being the cause of his death.

I aimed at the legionnaire. He seemed not to have moved at all from the fortified foxhole where he sat, waiting and watching for more victims. How could I get him? Then it dawned on me that Beni's rifle was much better than mine. I reached for it on the bottom of the trench where it had fallen. I lifted it, concentrating on my aim with all the energy and drive I could muster. I could see the legionnaire's face. Was he laughing at me? I could only see his eyes and nose; the rest of his face was protected by the foxhole. But I was certain he was smiling, jeering at my inability to get him.

I prayed again. This time for victory over my personal enemy, that particular legionnaire, whom I had never met or talked to. As I aimed, I also saw Ben's bleeding shoulder and Ahmed's stare of death. I prayed to the Jewish God for revenge and fired one bullet. It hit the legionnaire between the eyes and he died instantly. I was triumphant. I had won the no man's land between us.

Help arrived shortly and Beni was evacuated. I scrambled over the trench and ran the short distance to my former enemy's position. The prize of battle awaited me: the Bren submachine gun with lots of ammunition, more than I had ever seen at the front.

Near the gun lay the dead legionnaire, a surprised look on his face. Beside him was a pile of personal belongings he must have looked at from time to time while lying in wait for his victims. I reached down to look and saw a photograph of his wife and three children, inscribed in Arabic, "With love to Daddy." I was speechless. Tears welled up in my eyes and spilled over on to the dead legionnaire's uniform as I stood over him. I was never quite sure of the meaning of those tears. Was I crying for my enemy, I wondered, or for Poor Ahmed the mule? Were those tears for Beni's wound, or for myself, who had become a murderer in the struggle for life and survival?

XI

The Changing of the Guard

*

*L*ife moves in a never-ending cycle taking its own natural course. The predictable seasons move from spring to summer to fall to winter and back to spring again. Sometimes we are surprised, of course. In the middle of fall, an unexpected snowstorm can hit, but then the normal pattern of fall reasserts itself. In my life, too, there have been cycles as well as unforeseen events. Each has shaped my destiny, for better or for worse.

We won the battle against the Arab states that tried to destroy Israel at birth, but we weren't really able to win the war. The shadow of Arab hostility to the Jewish presence in the "Sea of Arabia" may never be eliminated, a fact which to this day shapes the personal destiny of Israelis.

In 1948 the task of rebuilding a nation from a hodgepodge of people seemed impossible. Survivors of concentration camps now lived side by side with Yemenite immigrants who had come from a completely different, still ancient, world. The "common" language, Hebrew, was not so common. Languages and traditions of hundreds of different groups had to meld. The Biblical land of "milk and honey" was all but destroyed and the harsh climate and terrain made reconstruction difficult.

I returned home to Papa from my reserve duty at the front. Our orange grove was neglected and overgrown, but still standing. Hyman, now grey and quite old, still brayed every morning like an alarm clock. But this bray was softer and more dignified. His faithful companion, Dummkopf, still kept close to his side, but she was no longer playful. Papa, too, had mellowed. Although less stubborn, he was just as impractical as ever and still only barely making a living. But it was good to be home and together again.

But it was not for long. I was soon drafted into the Army. The need for soldiers was acute given the fragile nature of the armistice. So Papa was left alone again. I came home on leave whenever I could, to help out and to provide some company. I was always full of stories and loved to sit outside talking after the work was done. Papa was a willing audience! He loved to hear about my life in the military. He was thrilled when I selected the Air Force for my military service once I made it through boot camp. For Papa, a Jewish Air Force was like a dream come true. It meant that Israel had become a real nation.

Gradually, he began to tell me more details of his youth as a Zionist revolutionary in Russia. Once, in Odessa, he had climbed a church tower as some of the townspeople gathered to prepare another pogrom against the Jews. He threw a bomb from the tower which killed a great number of those gathering and wounded scores of others.

"I escaped during the confusion, making my way to the port where a waiting ship smuggled me out of the country. That was the last pogrom in Odessa! I stopped them," he told me proudly.

There were stories of his life in Vienna as a leading Socialist party member. Also tales of our first years in Israel from a perspective I had rarely ever understood as a child. Over the years, many of his friends from Odessa and Vienna had come to Israel and now held high positions in the government. With eyes glowing and an excited voice, he spoke with pride of their accomplishments and the great accomplishments of others in the Zionist movement for which he had worked so hard. I hardly recognized him. Although I had heard many of the stories of his exploits before, I knew he was telling me everything because he now thought of me as a man, an equal, and my heart swelled with pride.

On one of my visits, Papa awakened me early in the morning.

"Hyman is dead, Yehuda. He died in his sleep." I dressed quickly and ran to the place where Hyman always stood. He was lying down, not moving. Tears welled up as my thoughts wandered back through the years we had spent together. That donkey was part of my life; not just a beast of burden, but a closer friend than many of my human companions.

"I will call the rendering plant, Yehuda," Papa shouted from the door, "They'll be happy. Hyman should produce a lot of glue!"

"Glue!" I shouted, "No, no no! No rendering plant for my Hyman!" I was horrified at the thought and furious at my father for his insensitivity. "I will bury Hyman myself."

So I spent the morning digging his grave near a big orange tree, overlooking the valley, on the land that he worked for so many years. As I write this I realize that he has now turned to dust. But his memory is with me and still vivid.

✳ ✳ ✳

Life continued. My visits to Papa became sporadic as I entered into my Air Force career with enthusiasm and intensity. The Israeli Air Force wasn't much of a force at the time. We were long on ambition and very short on planes and training. Our planes were mostly an assortment of World War I German and British fighter planes. Our pilots were mostly well-intentioned volunteers, some were mercenaries and soldiers of fortune. A good number of them spoke no Hebrew, but most spoke some English or German.

My brother Dov was Chief Administrative Officer of the Air Force. Because of my ability to speak German and a little English, he assigned me to security duty, to help watch over our "foreign legions" making sure there were no spies or enemy sympathizers among those volunteers. For my "spare" time, he assigned to me the position of Chief Cultural Officer. For this job I received an additional eight dollars a month and my triple sergeant's stripes.

Of the two positions, the security job, naturally, was much more important to the Air Force, and fairly difficult for me. The cultural officer's job, on the other hand, was a lot of fun. One of my first duties was to open our library. We had received a mountain of donated books, all of which had to be sorted. They ranged from books on Chinese cooking, written in Italian, to Karl Marx's *Das Kapital* written in German. Fortunately, there were also many books on Jewish and Arab culture and history. These were constantly in demand as the immigrant soldiers struggled to learn about Israel, the Middle East and the context of the current struggle.

It was in the library that I first met my future wife, who would be my life's companion for thirty-four years. For me it was love at first sight. She had beautiful black eyes and hair, and deep olive skin; her smile was so innocent!

To get her attention I began to give orders in a loud voice to my assistant librarian. I wanted her to know right away how important I was! When I was sure she had heard enough to get the idea, I went over to her.

"Hi, Chayelet [soldier]. Would you like to go swimming in the sea this afternoon? I can get you on the truck. No charge either, since I am the one who makes the arrangements. Several other girls are going, too, so you won't be alone."

She looked at me with those big black eyes and that endearing smile. "Well, I would love to go, but I am from Jerusalem and have never been to the ocean to swim. I don't even know how."

"Oh, don't worry. I will take care of you, and teach you how to swim in no time!" This was perfect, I thought. I would be able to show off my prowess as a swim instructor and get very close to the object of my affections while doing so!

An hour later we were on the way to the ocean at Jaffa. There were no cabins at the beach: the girls had some problems changing underneath their big beach towels, which kept blowing around. Watching from afar, my friends and I were most interested in those windy revelations.

Finally my "dream boat" was ready, stepping out from behind the towel in a borrowed, one-piece blue suit that made her look even more attractive than before. We walked toward the water. The sea and I were both strangers to her, and she was just a little frightened, though trying not to show it. I took her hand to help her through the surf at the shore out to the calmer water.

"Now, lie down across my arms, and I'll show you the breast stroke." With some trepidation she followed instructions, and as I supported her stomach she practiced the stroke. As she got the hang of it, I guided her into deeper water until finally she couldn't touch bottom. Since she couldn't stand, and still could not swim, there was no alternative for her other than to hold on to me.

This was heavenly, I could feel her breasts against my chest as she hung on for dear life. I had my arms around her, hugging her as if I had known her considerably longer than the two hours that had passed since I'd first seen her in the library. I kissed her on the cheek, without asking permission.

"Please take me back!" she said sternly, but there was a little twinkle in her eye and a shy smile on her lips, and she didn't object when I gave her another hug. I felt like a combination of lifeguard and victor in battle.

Slowly we moved toward the shore. I was reluctant to end this session and used every opportunity to move her closer to me and to change our positions a little so I could feel her body against mine. I expected a well deserved slap on the face once she was safely ashore, but maybe my sad Bogart look (by now, well practiced) had hypnotized her. Instead of a slap, she grabbed my hand and told me how much she had enjoyed her first time in the ocean, even though she had been scared to death!

The sun was like a giant fireball in the sky as we rode back together in the truck. Back at the base, after a falafel and a coffee, we went to the evening movie. It was "Gone With the Wind," the perfect romantic movie to top off a romantic day. We sat in "lovers row," the last row in the cinema, holding hands and kissing. Her feminine defenses were down after our afternoon of closeness in the ocean! We left the movie before it ended, to finish our evening under the stars on a nearby sandy beach.

My new girlfriend's family and tradition were very different from mine. I was European. She was Middle Eastern. Her mother, who had come to Israel on a donkey from Egypt, still spoke only Arabic. I belonged to the middle class. Her family was very poor and lived in Jerusalem in an area severely damaged during the 1948 war. Their house was surrounded by half-ruined buildings not yet reconstructed. It was about 150 years old, made of reddish Jerusalem limestone with a mosque-like dome in the center. It had no gas, no running water, no indoor toilet, no electricity and was cold and drafty in the winter, humid in summer.

My family was small, consisting now of just Dov, Papa and me, while she came from a greatly extended family. Her six brothers and sisters and their children (one brother alone had fourteen of them!) were always visiting at their mother's house. I will never forget the first time I met them all. As I walked into the big, high-domed living room I felt like one hundred pairs of black eyes were boring into me! They looked at me, with my blue eyes and fair skin, as if I had come from another planet. But in a few moments we were all laughing and at ease together. Their family spirit was wonderful and they went out of their way to make me feel at home — no, like a king. *Umi* (Mom), who was just about as wide as she was tall, brought out some *salata matbucha* (a cooked salad which became a favorite of mine forever) and my high school Arabic was put to the test as we talked away the afternoon.

Our cultural and family differences were of little concern to me at this point: I was in love and very determined. With the help of my brother, my chaticha (girlfriend) became my secretary in the cultural office. She wasn't really trained for this, but she definitely made every effort to do well!

One of the duties of the cultural officer was to take care of the volunteer performing artists who came to entertain the troops and to play host at their shows. It was fairly easy to get pretty big name stars, because at the time just about everybody who was anybody in Hollywood donated two weeks a year to causes in support of Israel, which often included coming to Israel to entertain. When they arrived at our base, my job was to make sure they were happy, had their whims catered to, and that they arrived on time for their evening performance.

One day, Danny Kaye walked into my office and saluted me as if I were a general.

"I understand I am supposed to present myself to you for tonight's performance. Well, here I am, Sir!"

"Sir, it is my honor to have you here," I said, jumping to my feet and struggling to think and speak in English. I was startled at being spoken to with such respect by this famous star! "Please let me know if there is anything you need while you are here. It's my job to see that you are well taken care of."

"I doubt if I will need much, Sergeant. But could you show me the stage where I will be performing tonight? I need a little rehearsal time more than anything else."

That afternoon and evening are still memorable for me. I was a nervous wreck as I introduced Mr. Kaye at the show. He was by far the most famous artist I had ever had to introduce.

His performance was wonderful. There were two thousand soldiers watching. Many of them couldn't speak English, and he couldn't speak more than ten words of Hebrew, but there was a chemistry that enabled him to reach out and move the audience to sing along — songs he knew and songs he tried to learn from us. The closeness between audience and performer was glorious.

Finally, in the wee hours of the morning, the chauffeur arrived to take Mr. Kaye to his reserved suite at the Hilton Hotel. He looked at me with tired blue eyes.

"Sergeant, I really would prefer to sleep here in a soldiers' tent with the rest of you. Just one night, I want to feel like a true soldier of Israel."

I was touched. I had the arrangements made and he slept that night with ordinary soldiers. Danny Kaye was probably the most down-to-earth celebrity I have ever met. His memory stays with me as much for that reason as for his impressive grace and talent.

There were other performers who stick in my mind for other reasons. An American opera singer, for example, who arrived in a state of extreme agitation, with a chauffeur assigned to her by the Army and with her two miniature schnauzers. The dogs immediately began to bark ferociously at all the uniformed soldiers, and at me in particular.

"I absolutely cannot perform tonight, Sergeant. My babies have no food! The airline left their special dog food in New York. Without it they will starve! They won't eat anything else!"

"I shall telex New York immediately. They'll put the suitcase on the very next plane, I'm sure," I said, trying to calm her down, "In the meantime, your dogs can eat the food our soldiers eat."

"Ugh," remarked the army driver, "That stuff isn't fit for dogs! It will do them in for sure!"

It took some doing after that remark, but finally the singer agreed to perform, provided I personally took care of her "babies" and got them some decent, non-Air Force food.

Then there was the male vocalist, extremely famous, who requested that I find him a new virgin every night to entertain him after he entertained the troops. To my amazement, I had no trouble finding volunteers during the two weeks of his stay!

All my efforts in support of the visitors did not go unnoticed by the high command. Soon I was given my own private room on the top of the apartment complex at our Jaffa compound. As chief administrative officer, my brother had a whole apartment, but that didn't bother me. A room of my own was all I needed to begin entertaining pretty young women soldiers. Of course, my principal guest was my lovely little secretary. We spent many afternoons lying on my couch listening to Italian music together, though neither of us understood the lyrics. I put my arm around her and caressed her, whispering, *"Ti voglio bene* [I love you]," the one Italian phrase I knew.

※ ※ ※

Although my duties and girlfriend kept me very busy, I still went to visit my father at least once a week. He was lonely and often told me how much he wished I would stop by more frequently. But the chances to get away were few and far between.

Then one afternoon in October of 1950, as the first autumn winds were beginning to blow through the citrus trees, a meeting which I had expected to take all evening was canceled. I decided to hurry home and see Papa. For some reason, I had a feeling that it was very important I go right away. I had no money for the bus that week, so I set out hitchhiking.

I was alone with no attractive girl to get a driver's attention, so I wasn't so lucky getting a ride. I trudged along for quite awhile before I got a ride to the outskirts of my village. I stopped for a quick falafel before walking the final stretch, and I finally arrived about ten o'clock. It was pitch dark on the road up to the house. The door was unlocked but none of the petrol lights were on. When I got one of the lamps going, I could see that Papa had been reading a history of Russia. It lay open on the table.

The house was clean. The bed was made. Where was Papa? I had a feeling something was wrong; he always retired at nine, since he was such an early riser. I opened the door and listened to the voices of night; hyenas called in the distance. Fireflies were riding the night winds.

As my eyes and ears adjusted to the dark, I became aware of the sound of water, like rain. The irrigation system! Odd that it was on so late. Not a star was in the sky that night, but I knew the way to the shut-off valve. I still remember the strong smell of the lemon trees.

As I reached the main valve and bent to turn it off, I stumbled over something massive. Papa. Dead, with the wrench for turning off the valve clutched in his fist. I couldn't move. I could hardly breathe. Finding him so unexpectedly, his death so undreamed of!

I pulled myself together, worked the wrench free from his stiff hand and turned off the water. Then I lay down in the grass next to Papa, looking up to the dark sky for some sign of his soul escaping without a good-bye or blessing, leaving just his cold body on the earth. That night I thought my search was in vain, but I have come to realize that I carry a piece of his soul with me.

A while later, I made my way to our neighbor Chaim's house.

"Papa is dead," I yelled from the front gate. "Call the police and ambulance and come and help, please."

Soon the night was illuminated with the policemen's spotlights, shining down on my father as he lay on the land he had worked with love and dedication for so many years. After the ambulance left, I went to Chaim's and called the newspaper so the funeral announcement would appear in the morning edition, just making the deadline.

✳ ✳ ✳

The funeral was late in the afternoon. Blacky, the same horse who had pulled my mother's funeral wagon, took my Papa now. There were scores of people present. Cabinet ministers, labor leaders, the future President of Israel and, most important, the *amcha,* the people, many of whom I had never met. I never realized how important my Papa had been to so many people. To me, he had always seemed a bit lost in Israel.

The coffin was draped with the flag of Israel. The ceremony was only minimally religious, on my orders and according to what Papa would have wished. There was only one eulogy, given by Papa's dear friend, Mendel Singer.

"Today we say, 'Shalom,' to our dearest comrade, Pinchas. He lived and died for the blessed land of Israel. A man of few words and many deeds. Early in his life he single-handedly stopped pogroms in Odessa with his daring attack from the church tower. Later, he withstood humiliation and defeat from the Nazis, bringing his family to this land to begin again. Here, too, he struggled for the cause of Israel. Pinchas died with a smile on his face, knowing his mission was accomplished."

The grave was closed. The mourners streamed past, leaving the customary little stone at the graveside and dedicating a personal moment to their departed friend.

I cried softly as the crowd dispersed. Soon only Dov, Moishe the balegula and I were left. Once more, I stroked Blacky's beautiful head. His mane had turned white with age.

"You know, that was Blacky's last funeral," Moishe said. "We got a funeral car to take his place." I cried in earnest. It was the end of an era: the changing of the guard.

XII

Off to Veterinary School

*

*I*t was the fall of 1951. The fresh, salty sea breeze blew on my face. The flag on the mast of *Jerusalem,* the flagship of Israel, fluttered gaily above us. We were in the port of Haifa, standing at the foot of the gangway leading to the ship. The whole family was there to wish me farewell and good luck in "Spaghetti Land." I was off to Italy, to study veterinary medicine at the University of Pisa.

Soon after my Papa's death, I received my discharge from the Air Force, got married, and returned home to take care of the *pardess.* Papa's closest friends, however, encouraged me to continue my schooling. "Your Mom always wanted you to be a doctor, Yehuda. You have the talent, don't stay here with the orange trees all your life."

"But I don't have the money!" I replied. "And my wife is already pregnant! How can I afford to go to school?"

"Don't be so short sighted!" everybody said. "You can move to Jerusalem and study pre-med at Hebrew University. Live with your wife's family. That won't cost you anything. We will help you rent the place here and you can use the funds to pay for the tuition."

And so it was arranged. We moved into my mother-in-law's home, and I began my studies. In my heart, I knew I would never be an M.D. There was no way I could afford the ten years of study it would take. Besides, my heart was not in it. I remembered how my mother suffered all those years, when her doctors could do very little for her. I didn't think I could take it, to watch my patients suffer as she had, without being able to help them live or end their suffering.

My love for animals made it natural for me to move from human to veterinary medicine. The only problem was that there was no veterinary school in Israel, so I would have to go abroad. Deciding where was easy: the closest, cheapest, and easiest place to be admitted was Italy. While I finished my first year in Jerusalem, I applied at several Italian schools and finally selected the University of Pisa, mainly because I knew there were several other Israeli students there already.

So here I was, on the dock, preparing to embark.

I was going alone. Although I had no difficulty obtaining a visa, the foreign currency allotment assigned by the Israeli government at the time was barely enough for one person. So my wife and baby would have to remain home until I figured something out.

The port was crowded and noisy as people gathered in groups to see their friends and relatives off. Porters pushed through the crowd with luggage, children were running, people hugged and kissed and cried. Arms were waving and messages shouted into the wind as people boarded the ship, leaving their friends ashore.

The ship's piercing whistle blew, and made the baby cry. I picked her up to comfort her, swinging her up onto my shoulders.

"Let's play our favorite donkey-riding game, Fafa," I said, letting out an authentic donkey bray. This almost always got her laughing again. But not this time! Instead I felt a warm stream of fluid down my neck and back. I was soaked clear down to my new pants!

Everyone began to laugh.

"Look on the bright side!" said Dov, "It could have been Number Two!"

I was not amused. In the midst of this my sister-in-law, Eva, began to sing, "Addio patria mia," from *Aida* at the top of her voice, causing every-one to stare at us. We were quite a sight: plump, operatic Eva, screaming Fafa, well-soaked Yehuda, with my wife and Dov laughing so hard they were sobbing.

By now, Eva had moved on in her repertoire to "Dolce Aida." A little short, slightly plump but very elegantly dressed lady, with the smallest dog I have ever seen straining at his leash, stopped to listen. She was obviously Italian and an opera appassionata.

"*Brava,*" she exclaimed, rushing up to give Eva a big kiss on the cheek. "You are as good as Maria Callas!" This was stretching the truth, but nevertheless it made Eva swell with pride. The pride expanded even more when the woman introduced herself as a contessa (a countess). Such praise from nobility!

Meanwhile, I was getting the royal treatment from the contessa's doggy. He was jumping all over me, probably attracted by the smell which now permeated my shirt and pants.

"A good omen for a veterinarian!" smirked Dov.

As I reached the top of the gangway, I noticed the contessa and the ship's captain engaged in heated conversation. Strudel, the dog, was barking furiously at the captain, who kept pointing toward the deck where Strudel had left a runny brown deposit. The contessa continued shouting. When I moved closer, Strudel ran happily over to me. I reached down and picked him up and he became very calm. The captain looked relieved. The contessa looked grateful.

"How long have you known this dog?" asked the captain in Hebrew.

"About five minutes, but I'm a doctor of veterinary medicine," I said, conveniently leaving out the words, "or will be in five years."

"*Veterinario!*" exclaimed the contessa, who picked up on the Hebrew. "Oh, Captain," she pleaded in a mixture of Italian and English, "My Strudel is really sick and needs care. Nothing is more important! Would you please move the doctor to a cabin next to mine? That way I shall know he will be available whenever Strudel and I need him!"

The captain seemed amused that the contessa was ready to pay three times my ticket price to move me from the cheapest three-bunk room to a first-class cabin.

"Some dog!" he said to me in Hebrew, with a sly look. Without even waiting for my consent, he had the porter whisk away my bags to first class.

"*Grazie mille, signor dottore,*" smiled the countess. I returned the smile, flattered by the use of the term "Doctor," unearned though it was, and also unsure of what I was getting myself into.

As I stood up, straightening myself, I was suddenly struck by a wooden crutch which came crashing down on the deck from behind me. I turned and saw a beautiful blonde woman sprawled on the deck where she had slipped.

"Are you hurt?" I asked, lifting her up. She held on to my arm as I returned her crutch to her. I could see that one of her legs was atrophied, probably from polio.

"*Toda rabah, Adoni,*" she said in thanks. Her smile made me melt. She walked away toward the lower deck entrance, her long hair blowing in the wind.

The ship was now freed from its moorings. From the rail I could still see my family. Gradually, they, the port and the city of Haifa faded from sight. Tears came to my eyes as I watched Mt. Carmel in the distance topped with one golden cloud illuminated by the setting sun. I was leaving my adopted homeland for the first time since arriving as a frightened little refugee. Soon the rolling fog enveloped the shoreline and I realized I was all alone on the deck.

Later, I ended up in the lounge, where a terrific quintet was playing wonderful Italian tunes for ballroom dancing. Across the room I saw the blonde woman who had fallen on deck just before our departure. She motioned me to join her table.

The evening passed quickly. We spoke of our families, my plans for study in Pisa, her job in the Israeli Air Force and the advanced telecommunications classes she was being sent to take in Rome.

The few days it took for the crossing passed quicky and most pleasantly; finally one morning we docked in the busy and certainly noisiest port I have ever seen: Naples. As I said goodbye to the contessa, the tall Italian who had carried her bags when I first saw her appeared from out of nowhere. He wisked her away with Strudel barking goodbye and scampering along behind.

"Lost your first client, Doctor?" laughed Dina, creeping up from behind.

"Do you have any need for my veterinary services, young lady?" I replied in mock seriousness. "I am not quite yet a doctor, but perhaps we could discuss this over tea. . . ."

From Naples, I found my way to the railroad station and boarded a train for the last leg of my trip to my destination in Pisa.

XIII

Migliarino and the Two-Headed Calf

*

I stood on the train station platform in Pisa. Now I had to begin the work I was sent to do: become a veterinarian in earnest. I had to learn Italian. I needed a place to live and a job. I had very little money and I knew no one. With these tasks in mind, I collected my bags and walked into town.

It was still very early. The bells were ringing their morning songs from the church towers. The town seemed almost magical to me. I was fascinated by the musicality of the Italian language, as people greeted each other on the street or called down from their windows to their departing husbands and children. The town was not yet rebuilt after the damages caused by the war, which were masked by the Italians' cheerfulness and love for life. I walked through the ancient arches of the medieval city, and crossed the river Arno to reach the center of the old town. With the few words of Italian I knew, I asked directions to the synagogue.

Some men were leaving as I approached the massive fortress of a building; they directed me to Rabbi Attilio's study, where I found him poring over books and papers. He was very cordial and made me feel welcome immediately.

"There are a few other Israelis in Pisa," said the Rabbi. "Most of them are studying to be veterinarians. I think the best thing for you would be to get to know them right away. They will be able to give you good advice. At this time of day, you should find them at a cafe near the Piazza dei Miracoli. They have become very Italian," he laughed with a twinkle in his eye. "You will see. We Italians work only when we have to. The rest of the time we talk and enjoy life. Look for Avram. He will be playing his accordion and singing with whatever group he can gather around him."

I found my way to the piazza and was so overcome with the beauty of the *Duomo*, the cathedral, and the Leaning Tower — gleaming, dazzling white in the morning sun — I almost missed the Israeli contingent. They were just leaving as I arrived at the cafe. The leader of the group, Avram, was tall and dark and looked very Italian. As the Rabbi had said, he was playing his accordion and singing a medley of folk songs at the top of his lungs — in Italian, then Russian, then Hebrew. He looked like the Pied Piper as he strolled out of the cafe followed by his entourage.

"So you are one of the new students from Israel we have heard about," the group chorused as I introduced myself. "You will love Italy!" Then they bombarded me with questions.

"I thought there were two new Israeli students. Where is the other one?"

"He's coming later," I replied.

"What's the news from Israel?"

They interrupted before I had a chance to answer.

"Do you speak Italian?" "How much is your foreign exchange allotment?" "Do you sing?"

"Quiet," Avram said to them, taking charge. Then he turned to me. "You have only one month before school starts. You must learn Italian. Follow my advice and it will be easy for you. Go to the movie house early in the morning. Stay the whole day and see the same movie over and over again. By the end of the day you will understand the plot and the words will start to make sense."

Avram had lots of other advice which he dispensed in quite a superior manner, definitely not to my liking. But his advice on the movie seemed sensible and I took it. He was right. After a day, I not only understood the movie, I had learned Italian intonation and pronunciation and had developed a sense of confidence that made learning the language much easier. By the time my friend Charlie arrived from Israel two weeks later, I was doing really well. Of course, I told Charlie the all-day movie house method, and he used it too, although he didn't need it as much as I had; he was originally from Romania, and Romanian and Italian are sister languages.

Charlie and I had met in Jerusalem at the Hebrew University. He also wanted to become a vet and we had become fast friends, sharing many mutual interests, including our love of animals. When Charlie arrived, I moved from my single small room in a boarding house into a much larger room which Charlie and I shared with a Greek student.

The very next morning we woke up to find our roommate missing, along with all our cash. This was a real disaster! Our next monthly allotment from home was not due for ten days and we didn't have enough to even buy bread.

"We'll find a job," Charlie announced, undaunted, "and one that includes room and board."

Borrowing the newspaper from our landlady, he scoured it for possibilities. He came across an advertisement for a *tuttofare,* or "do-everything," for one of the local priests. It included room and board.

"Perfect!" he cried, "I will go immediately. Perhaps he will also know of a similar job for you."

He returned a short time later. "My God, Guido," Charlie exclaimed using my adopted Italian name. "You won't believe what that priest had in mind when he said he was looking for a *tuttofare!* The man is homosexual! And he made no bones about the fact that among my more important duties would be to provide sexual favors. I would rather starve than take that job!"

Well, we didn't starve. But for the next few weeks we were almost always hungry. With the assistance of the Rabbi, we obtained a small loan from local Jewish community funds to tide us over until our money arrived. The rabbi also told us about the possibility of work at an agricultural farm called Cevoli. There would be no pay, but there was supposed to be room and board. Cevoli was a farm set up by a wealthy Jewish-Italian professor to help train teenage Italian Jews to be farmers in preparation for immigration to Israeli *kibbutzim.* The professor had gone to teach at the Hebrew University in Jerusalem and while he was there he decided to spend his life helping to foster the immigration of Italian Jews. So he founded Cevoli as a sort of training camp.

"The farm needs Hebrew teachers as well as instructors in agriculture. I know the manager will be delighted to have your services," said the Rabbi. "I cannot go with you, but here is a letter which will introduce you to the manager. Why not take the Pontedera bus this afternoon?"

Two hours later we arrived at Cevoli. The sun was setting as we descended from the bus into the Italian countryside, its last golden rays touching the vast green fields which surrounded us. Being used to dry, arid Israel, the greenness of the Italian vineyards and hills overwhelmed us.

As the rabbi had expected, the manager was indeed glad to have us. He was proud of the work he was doing and excited by the idea of preparing young men and women to immigrate to Israel, their spiritual homeland. In truth, the teenagers were more interested in teenage pursuits than in agricultural ones and their attention span for learning Hebrew and Israeli customs was minimal. As far as Charlie and I were concerned, the room and board turned out to be almost non-existent. We slept on lumpy mattresses on the cold floor of the ancient farmhouse. The food was meager and frequently awful. We were always hungry.

One night, after a particularly terrible dinner, Charlie and I wandered into the spindly garden.

"Maybe we'll find a tomato or two left on the vine," I said, "Even a green one would taste good!" The garden was not well kept because of lack of interest on the part of the farm's principal workers, so we didn't hold out too much hope of finding something edible.

"Here's one!" cried Charlie, "And there are two more next to the chicken coop. What luck!" As I walked toward the chicken coop to retrieve the tomatoes, I heard the unmistakable sound of a hen about to lay an egg.

"Charlie," I called. "How about some eggs to go with the tomatoes?" We entered the coop and started looking through the nests of hay where the chickens did their laying. No eggs. Our disappointment was keen. We had already eaten those eggs in our imagination!

We turned and eyed the hens. Which one was it that was about to lay? We would wait.

"It's this one, Charlie. You'll see. Just hold on." Minutes passed. No more cackling. Nothing.

"The hen has decided to lay tomorrow," said Charlie, challenging my knowledge of chickens.

"Maybe so, but let's try to persuade her to hurry up." I picked her up with one hand holding her wings together behind her back. With the other hand, I squeezed her rear to push the egg out, but gently so as not to break the egg inside.

"One, two . . . three!" I counted and out popped the egg into Charlie's waiting hand. Charlie was astounded. Of course, I had never told him about the hundreds of chickens that I had handled in the past, both dead and alive.

"Anybody who can squeeze an egg out of a chicken's behind will never starve," laughed Charlie as we divided the raw egg over our tomatoes and sat down to satisfy our hunger.

When our school started, Charlie and I commuted by bus into Pisa from the farm, a distance of some thirty miles. The combination of bad sleeping arrangements, terrible food, uninterested kids and a long commute soon proved too much for us. Our "free room and board" just wasn't worth it. We moved to Migliarino, a small village closer to the University. From there we could ride bicycles to our classes and we found more than adequate lodging with a delightful old farmer named Bartolini. He gave Charlie a small room in the farmhouse and introduced me to *signor* Gino, who helped me move into a building across the road. Shortly thereafter I sent for my wife and baby, using the money I had saved during my stay at Cevoli to pay for their passage.

Our little apartment in Migliarino was clean, but we had no running water. We had to bring it in buckets from the public fountain some distance away. And we were poor! The meager allotment was even more meager now that there were three of us. Fortunately, my wife was a magician with cooking. She could do wonders with bruised or damaged potatoes, artichokes, corn, and with cheap cuts of meat like beef heart.

She couldn't speak the language, so I did most of the shopping when she first arrived. At that time, I was a fanatic for saving money. There was always the threat of war in Israel and the chance that our funds would be cut off. I was determined that we should save half of the little sum we got each month. I became an expert in finding the cheapest buys for everything, taking advantage of my wife's ignorance of Italian to purchase cuts of meat she would never have dreamed of buying, then telling her they were something else! Blood sausage, for example, became liverwurst.

Blood sausage was the cheapest meat around, but it was made from blood and pig fat. No observant Jew would ever consider eating blood sausage. And although she had become considerably less observant than when she first married me, my wife would never have tolerated it had she known what it really was. But we were so poor that I decided to bypass her religious scruples and buy it anyway. I have to admit I was a little embarrassed to ask the butcher for it the first time, so I ignominiously attempted to conceal my Jewishness, taking great pains to tell the butcher, in my still halting Italian, that I was Australian. I don't know whether he really believed me, especially in view of the fact that in little Migliarino everybody knew everything about everyone. But at least he played along.

Thanks to my lack of conviction and my wife's cooking prowess, we enjoyed blood sausage prepared in every possible way until she learned enough Italian to start shopping on her own.

"Ah, *Signora,* welcome!" the butcher exclaimed upon her first visit to his shop. "You are the Australian's little wife, aren't you? He has told me so much about you, what a good cook you are. . . ."

"Please sir," she said, confused by the Australian reference but assuming she had misunderstood the Italian, "I would like some liver sausage. I know my husband buys it from you all the time and that you give him a very good price."

"Liver sausage? No, no, *Signora,* he never buys liver sausage. He only buys blood sausage. He is one of my best customers for this. He says you are a genius at preparing it!"

Well, that was the end of our blood sausage days. My wife's willingness to accept my rather casual approach to religion and my ferocious devotion to saving money did not extend to consciously eating pork, even if it was the least expensive meat around.

✳ ✳ ✳

We settled into a routine. Charlie and I would bicycle to school every morning and every night after supper we would walk together for miles along the road leading out of the village, asking each other questions, Socrates style, preparing for our next day's classes or exams. Our only distraction were the prostitutes waiting for their customers along a tree-lined route nicknamed, on their account, the Via delle Belle Donne, the Street of the Pretty Women. "Good discount for students!" they would call to us as we walked by. But we weren't interested. We just kept walking and studying, becoming almost as much of an institution on that road as the ladies.

As a result of our efforts, Charlie and I became the best students in our class. The professors loved our dedication and devotion to their subjects, a devotion not shared by most of our Italian colleagues, who, although bright, generally preferred to play around with the girls, sing and have a good time, studying just enough to get by. The school was old-fashioned and mostly theoretical, with very little clinical experience to offer students.

Our first anatomy class consisted of a visit to the Veterinary Anatomical Museum in Milan, established by a former professor at the university who had spent his career developing a secret technique for the preservation of anatomical specimens of animals. Just about every kind of animal was on display, all dried and preserved, but looking fresh and natural.

I particularly remember that first visit to the museum. The variety of animals on display was amazing. We were awed by our professor's detailed anatomical knowledge of so many different creatures, and also by the fact that we, too, would be expected to learn the anatomy of over ten species! The hours flew by as we passed from mouse to fish, from chicken to horse, going through the museum listening to our instructor. At the conclusion of our tour, Professor Romboli looked at our serious, exhausted faces and at the reams of notes we had taken, and laughed.

"Ah, but the most interesting creature of all is yet to come!" he said. And there by the exit, staring at us out of a large jar, was the floating head, fully bearded, of the anatomy professor who had created the museum. The inscription on the jar read: "I dedicated my professional life to creating the displays in this museum, and they are all very dear to me. I have chosen to become a part of my life's work even in death."

✳ ✳ ✳

My first real "clinical" veterinary experience didn't involve the school at all. One night at about two o'clock in the morning, Charlie knocked on our door.

"Come quickly, Guido. Farmer Bartolini's cow is trying to calf and is having problems. He wants us to try to help." Charlie's landlord had always been extremely nice to both of us and we wanted to repay his kindness by helping him in any way we could.

Of course farmer Bartolini was far more knowledgeable than we were, having participated in hundreds of calf births, and Charlie and I were more than a little terrified when we discovered he really thought our few months of veterinary school meant we could do something he couldn't.

"I've been a farmer for forty years and never had such a case," he said as we entered the barn. He was half naked, bloodied and exhausted from trying to extract the calf. "The head and both front feet are out and still the calf is stuck! This is my best cow. I simply don't know what to do. Maybe there's something in those books you two are always reading that will help?"

Charlie was a better student than I, but had no practical experience at all. He turned to me. Summoning my "experience" from the birth of Dummkopf's baby and everything I could remember from the instructions Dr. Ellenberger had given me back then, I poured mineral oil over my hands and reached into the moaning cow's birth canal.

I soon found the problem, but could scarcely believe it. The calf had two heads!

"*Dio Santo!*" cried Farmer Bartolini, crossing himself and praying devoutly to his Catholic God to give his Jewish first year veterinary student neighbor the expertise to save his best cow.

"We will need to cut the second head off in the womb," I explained. "I don't know what else to do. It is placed on the neck and shoulders in such a way that it is lying sideways. I don't think there is any way for the calf to be born unless we sever the head." I looked at Charlie helplessly, knowing that neither one of us was ready for such a task.

"*Dio Santo! Dio Santo!*" repeated farmer Bartolini. "My best cow. This is an impossible job. *Dio Santo! Dio Santo!*"

"Well, we must try," said Charlie firmly. "Otherwise the cow will die for sure. There is no time to bring a veterinarian from Pisa. Guido has worked on animals on his farm in Israel. He will do his best for you."

Later I learned that there was a special instrument for this type of surgery, but that night all we had that was small and sharp enough was my Swiss army knife. With Charlie at my side and Bartolini repeating, *"Spirito Santo! Santa Maria! Dio abbi pietà!"* I pushed the protruding head and legs back into the birth canal and began the tedious, bloody work. A slip of the knife and I would have punctured the wall of the womb and caused the cow's death. Slowly, slowly, I cut. The cow was moaning and her contractions continued, hampering my ability to make the amputation.

Finally, the head was off. Blood was gushing everywhere as I struggled to maneuver the severed head into position to pull it out. At last I pulled it free, losing my balance and tumbling backward on the floor. As I lay there exhausted, the cow had a violent contraction and the entire calf was expelled like a projectile on top of me. Farmer Bartolini grabbed a large butcher knife and severed the calf's other head to end its agony.

"Dio Santo!" he yelled. I still cannot hear this phrase without thinking of that night. "Guido, that was a miracle. You will be a fantastic doctor," he said, helping me up from the floor, "Come, you must eat after this ordeal. My wife will fix you breakfast."

I looked down at my blood-covered clothes and body, feeling exhausted and ready to go back to bed, not to breakfast! But farmer Bartolini insisted. Charlie helped me wash up while Bartolini tended to his exhausted, but living, cow. Farmer Bartolini's wife prepared an enormous breakfast. It smelled so good that I forgot my tiredness and joined in *con gusto*.

"Signora, this is wonderful," I said. "My wife and I are so poor just now. We never eat this well!"

"You shall have half the calf, Guido, as my thank you and payment for your services," said Bartolini, "That will help improve your dinners!"

In fact our dinners were significantly improved long after the meat from the calf was gone. Bartolini recounted the night's events to practically everyone in the village. The complexity of the event, the monstrosity of the two-headed calf, and the extent of my veterinary prowess grew with each retelling. This was big news in Migliarino. Villagers began to stop by to talk about the famous two-headed calf and how I had managed to save Bartolini's cow, Gina, the record milk-producer of the village. Each time they brought fresh vegetables or fruit and sometimes a chicken for *"il dottore,"* as everyone now called me. Thanks to the two-headed calf, we ate very well indeed for the rest of the time we lived in Migliarino.

In a small way, the two-headed calf also helped lessen the unconscious anti-Semitism which many villagers harbored. Bartolini called the village priest in to exorcise the demon which had caused Gina's aberrant calf and most of the village came to watch the elaborate and mysterious ceremony. When it was over, Mrs. Bartolini spoke with the priest.

"Father, you must meet *il dottore* and provide your blessing on him for all he has done," she told him. "I know he is Jewish. But Our Lord must have been with him through this miraculous event. He is a wonderful man." Somewhat reluctantly, the priest crossed the road to our little apartment, accompanied by the Bartolinis and half of the village.

"This is our Jewish friend who saved our best cow, Father," Mrs. Bartolini introduced me.

"*Dottore*, I have heard of your great feat," he said. "We are all grateful for what you have done. Although you are Jewish, I shall pray for you and ask the Lord to bless you and make you a wonderful veterinarian." It was quite a sight, this group of Italian Catholics, brought up to hold the Jews responsible for the death of their Savior, standing in front of a poor Jewish student's door to hear their priest offer to include him in his prayers.

XIV

The Rabbi and His Pigeons

✻

Venice's Piazza San Marco is famous for its pigeons — they are almost as much of an attraction as the beautiful buildings which surround the square. Yet when I think of pigeons, it isn't the Piazza San Marco which comes to mind: it is Pisa, and Rabbi Attilio.

My wife and I had lived in Migliarino for about a year. I was supplementing our monthly allotment from home by selling eggs I purchased from local farmers. My customers were mainly my professors in Pisa. I didn't make as much money at this enterprise as I had in Israel, because there was no black market now and food was much more plentiful. Still, this "egg money" was a help. Charlie and I also did translations from German and English into Italian for several of our professors. But then, as now, professors were sadly underpaid and ours could barely afford to pay us for our work. We were getting by, but it wasn't easy. And there was rarely anything left over for fun, like going to the movies.

One day I was riding to school, balancing a basket of eggs on the handlebars of my noisy little *motorino,* when Avram, the unofficial leader of the Israeli student contingent in Pisa, called me aside.

"Guido, I have an idea for you."

Now Avram and I weren't really friends. He was wealthy, happy-go-lucky, and never had to work. He and the other Israeli students sometimes made fun of me and all my little jobs to earn money. I was a bit resentful of his carefree life and his reputation with the ladies. And I think he was a little jealous of my stature with the professors, which had risen above his because of my linguistic abilities and translations. But our love of music frequently brought us together socially and created a bond, despite our differences.

It was music, in fact, that made him call me over that morning as I rode to school.

"Rabbi Attilio needs someone to act as cantor from time to time and as a Sunday-school teacher," Avram advised me. "He's getting very old, you know, and his voice is almost gone. He asked me, but I'm not really interested. I think it would be perfect for you. You have a good voice and enough knowledge of our traditions to teach the kids. And you and your family could live for free in the synagogue in exchange for helping out the rabbi. You wouldn't have to take that long trip from Migliarino every day either."

How ironic. Could I, who had raised rabbits, never had a bar mitzvah, had eaten blood sausage and only rarely attended religious services be considered for such a position at all? On the surface, it seemed improbable.

In truth, I had always cherished the Jewish tradition, even if I did not observe all of its tenets. The Israeli school system had provided me with a strong background in our history and culture. My father and Rabbi Zager, who had helped me prepare for my ill-fated bar mitzvah, instilled in me a deep sense of pride in my heritage and a desire to continue learning about our people and culture. So I decided to make an appointment with Rabbi Attilio. After all, he had helped me many times since my arrival in Pisa — with the loan and with the farm at Cevoli. He was a very different sort of rabbi from the infamous Rabbi Dravin. I wanted to help him if I could.

On the date of my appointment with the rabbi, I parked my *motorino* alongside the fortress of the synagogue. It was difficult to recognize it as a temple. The beige walls blended in perfectly with those of the surrounding buildings. The only signs that these walls housed a synagogue were two small engraved Stars of David and a plaque in memory of the martyrs of the congregation who had died in World War II, either in concentration camps or fighting in the underground resistance.

There were scores of pigeons moving somewhat aimlessly about on the stone entryway. I jumped in surprise as they took off in startled flight when I approached. I guess I was a little nervous. Although I was very proud of my knowledge, I knew I really wasn't qualified for the job. The rabbi opened the side door of the two-hundred-year-old synagogue. He was a small, stooped and balding man.

"*Shalom,* Guido," he greeted me in a cordial, soft voice. He took both my hands. I still remember how pale and shrunken he was and, in contrast, how penetrating and demanding his eyes were.

"Please come in," he continued. "Let's talk and see if you can help me." My nervousness increased. I didn't know what he meant. Did he expect me to be knowledgeable in the traditional prayer chants of the

Jewish community of Pisa? Would it be enough that I spoke Hebrew and had the ability to teach it?

To my surprise, he didn't ask me anything about my knowledge of Judaism. This was not an interview in the traditional sense. It was a cry for help. Rabbi Attilio was in his eighties and very frail. As we entered the synagogue he put his hand on my shoulder.

"I simply cannot believe my good fortune that you are willing to come without pay, Guido. I can only offer you small quarters, a room which was originally the library. I am not sure it will be big enough for your family."

"We don't need much, Rabbi," I assured him, following slowly down the hall.

He opened the door and we entered a small room, the paint peeling from the walls. There wasn't much light, just a few rays of sun coming through the single tall window. Almost empty bookshelves lined most of the walls.

"Some library, eh, Guido?" Rabbi Attilio said in a sad voice. "The Nazis ransacked the synagogue. They took all the books they found here and burned them. But fortunately they didn't find the most valuable ones, and some even more valuable manuscripts! Come, I will show you." He shuffled to one wall and touched a lever concealed near one of the bookcases.

"Help me, Guido," he said. "I am not strong enough to do this by myself anymore. Pull with me on the lever until the wall starts to move."

To my amazement, as we pulled, the wall did indeed begin to move. Old hinges in the ceiling and floor creaked as we slowly turned the wall around. It was a hidden bookcase, not a flat wall! For centuries Jews had created these types of hiding places, false walls or removable floor boards, within synagogues — secret places to hide important documents or religious artifacts in times of danger or oppression. The hidden bookcase was crammed with books and papers.

"The Germans believed that books were a great enemy and took them away from people whenever they could." Rabbi Attilio had tears in his eyes as he remembered. "This hiding place had been here for a long time. Luckily, the congregation always kept its most valuable things here and on the day the Germans came, they were in a hurry. They didn't really look all that carefully. If they had, they might have realized that our best treasures were not among the things they destroyed. Let me show you." He reached for several ancient volumes, beautifully bound in hand-tooled leather. "Look, the Talmud Books, printed over a century ago. Our complete book of laws.

"And here, Guido, is one of the reasons why I need your help so badly." He pointed to boxes stuffed with yellowing and decaying paper. With a tremor in his voice and tears in his eyes, he said, "This is correspondence between my grandfather, Rabbi Luzzatto, truly a *zadik* (sage) and one of the most famous rabbis of Europe. What a story these letters tell of our people in Italy. The daily tribulations and dilemmas. . . . And the views of these famous rabbis on such wide ranging subjects! 'Is it acceptable to eat an egg laid on the Sabbath?' asks one of the letters, as if it were a life and death matter!

"The letters are truly wonderful to read, Guido. I have been trying to put them in order so that I could send them to the Hebrew University in Jerusalem. I know there are young scholars there who would appreciate the information. There are so few Jews left here but so many to remember! Half of the local Jews were killed in the war; besides, there is much intermarriage now and the children are brought up as Catholics." The rabbi paused for a long time. "My eyesight is failing. I can no longer see well enough to put the papers in order. With your help I can finish the job so this part of our history will not be lost."

"Of course I can help!" I exclaimed. "It would be an honor. Don't worry about the size of the room. It will be fine for us."

So it was arranged. A few days later, we said our good-byes to our friends in Migliarino and moved to our new quarters in the two-hundred-year-old synagogue in Pisa.

✳ ✳ ✳

"You really are sent from heaven, Guido," sighed Rabbi Attilio on our first real visit after we moved in. "As I told you, I am badly in need of help with my rabbinical duties. I just can't handle things anymore, and my voice has no strength to sing. Come, let me take you on a tour of the entire synagogue so you will know where everything is. And there is so much history here. I want you to know it all.

"Of course, the synagogue was built for a congregation of at least one thousand members," Rabbi Attilio said of the enormous building. "Now, there are fewer than one hundred left."

We moved from room to room with Rabbi Attilio recounting small episodes of history and pointing out features of particular interest. The sanctuary was in typical Sephardic style, with the pulpit in the center. Beautiful benches filled the center of the room, each with a brass plaque engraved with the name of the long-dead donor.

"The pulpit is rosewood, Guido, a gift from our brethren of the old Republic of Venice. Their mighty commercial fleet brought this precious wood from the Far East. I can still picture my grandfather chanting the *Kol Nidre* here to an awed congregation on Yom Kippur eve.

"And look at the intricate woodcarving in the lattice work on the *Ezrat Nashim*," he said, pointing to the women's seating area in the balconies on either side. The lattice permitted the women to view the ceremony below, but, in keeping with the Mediterranean tradition, it also screened them from the view of the men below. "Of course, now we only use the *Ezrat Nashim* on Yom Kippur, Guido. There are so few of us."

We moved back to the Eastern wall, facing toward Jerusalem and flanked on either end by two enormous bronze menorahs. Across the top of the wall were carved panels with lions, palm trees and pomegranates, the traditional Jewish symbols but no human images. In the center were carved the words, *"Ze beit ha Elohim* (This is the house of God)."

"The beautiful gold-stitched *parochet* (ornamental curtain) hanging above the holy arch was donated by Mrs. Cohen. She spent five years of her life embroidering it! The original one was destroyed by the Nazis when they ransacked the temple."

Rabbi Attilio's eyes lit up and he smiled as he spoke. "These American and Israeli flags you see on each side of the holy arch were given to us the day the Jewish Brigade and the American Jewish soldiers liberated us from the Nazis. It was like a miracle when these young soldiers showed up at our deserted synagogue. You cannot imagine what it meant to us."

We moved down the hallway.

"Here is where the Sunday school classes are held. You will have only six students. So few children," he sighed. "So many intermarriages now, so many Jewish children being raised as Catholics. . . ." he repeated to himself. *"Che tragedia* [what a tragedy]," he shook his head.

Finally we came to the rabbi's study. It was a small room with two windows looking out on a small courtyard filled with pigeons. The room was cluttered with mementos, books and papers, some old and some new, some valuable and some not. Rabbi Attilio walked over to the biggest window and opened it. Two pigeons immediately flew up from the courtyard and perched on the ledge. He stretched his hand through the wrought iron bars and held it out to the pigeons. They came over expectantly, cooing.

"My friends," the Rabbi said.

"Sit down, Guido," he said. "We must spend some time talking about the melodies you are to learn before we start on the music itself. You see, Italy was, until unification, a collection of small principalities and republics. The Jewish communities in each location developed different traditions of chants, which they have kept to this day. For example, if you attend services in Venice, Padua or Verona, you will find the prayers tend to be monotonous. But in Pisa our prayers have always been sung in operatic style.

"It will be a lot of work for you to capture the melodic style, Guido. Perhaps you should see a real opera before we begin to study. Yes, that's it! Tonight there is a performance of Verdi's *Nabucco* at the Teatro Verdi, just two doors down. It even has a Jewish theme, the exile of our people in Babylonia. Go to the performance, Guido, and listen carefully. Tomorrow, we will start working on the Friday night prayers and you will see how operatic music moved directly into the tradition of our synagogue."

The next day I returned to the rabbi's study in the late afternoon. As I entered, he was standing by the window with his hand extended through the bars to the two pigeons on the ledge.

"Ah, Guido, come in, come in. How was the opera? Did you listen carefully?"

"It was beautiful, rabbi," I replied, "I have not seen an opera since I was a young boy, when my mother took me on my donkey to see a performance of *La Belle Helène* in Kfar Saba. Last night, of course, was much more impressive. Overwhelming."

"Yes, and that is what your chants must be. You must bring out the *bel canto,* the operatic soul in our music, Guido. Come, stand here, next to me, and repeat each phrase. We will begin with the Friday night services. First the blessing of the Sabbath."

We worked for the next hour. The rabbi sang in his frail, but still beautiful voice, then I would try, usually managing only a few bars before he stopped me.

"No, no. Not like that. You must be stronger here, softer there. Try again." Or sometimes, "This phrase is the most important. Bring it out, Guido."

All the while, the two pigeons would sit on the ledge, sometimes cooing, but always watching. When we finished, the rabbi called me over to the window.

"Come meet your first critics, Guido. This is Bubale and this is Zubale. They have been my friends for many years. You must love animals since you study to be a veterinarian. I love these pigeons. All pigeons really. My father also loved the pigeons. I can't remember when we didn't have hundreds of them in the synagogue courtyard. Look at these below us. I think they are beautiful. Especially when they soar so freely up into the heavens. Look at them. They cover the courtyard, like a congregation coming to the temple."

He reached in his pocket and pulled out a packet of bread crumbs, tossing them on the ledge and then below into the courtyard. The flock began to chatter and moved about quickly, searching for the crumbs. Many flew up to the ledge, crowding around the rabbi's outstretched hand, tame enough to eat the bread crumbs from his palm.

"You know, Guido. We once had many more members in this congregation, many more members than the pigeons you see here in the courtyard. Now there are only a few left, but the number of pigeons continues unchanged after all these years. But these are just the sad musings of an old, old man. Don't listen to me. Come back tomorrow and we will work again." I left him feeding his pigeons.

✳ ✳ ✳

And so we continued for many weeks. By day, I attended school. By night, I studied into the wee hours of the morning in our cold little room, warming my feet next to an old and dangerous petrol heater, while my wife and little Fafa slept under layers of blankets. Late afternoons and early evenings were devoted to the rabbi; first helping him to organize his treasured papers and then going through the painstaking process of learning the Friday night services to his satisfaction. From the blessing of the Sabbath we moved to the Beracha, the consecration of the wine; on to *"Shalom Aleichem,"* the ushering in of the Sabbath Queen; and through all the prayers to the final one, the prayer of remembrance, the *Kaddish: Yitkadal Veyitkadash.*

The rabbi was right. The melodies were difficult to learn. Always, just as I began to feel I had mastered a phrase, Rabbi Attilio would interrupt.

"Listen again, Guido. Bring out the soul." And with his frail but still beautiful voice he would repeat the phrase the way it should be sung.

As always, the two pigeons Bubale and Zubale watched and cooed on the ledge just outside the window. After a few weeks, I was able to distinguish them from the others in the flock. They seemed to know just when we would begin our afternoon sessions; or perhaps they were just attracted to the glow of the study light on Rabbi Attilio's desk.

Was it my imagination, or did they especially like the *"Mizmor le David,"* praise for David, King of Israel? The rabbi patiently dispersed bread crumbs to them while listening to me practice. When we reached the *"Mizmor le David,"* they would almost always begin to coo while I chanted, as if to join me. When I was through, I would offer them bread crumbs too. But they would never eat from my hand. Only from Rabbi Attilio's.

Finally, I mastered all but the *Kaddish* prayer.

"Guido," said Rabbi Attilio impatiently one evening. "You must concentrate! I want you to be able to handle the complete service next Friday. This is important. You must be ready!"

Spurred by his insistence, I practiced long into the next few nights with him until he was finally satisfied that I knew all the prayers and chants for the service. On Sabbath night, I joined the rabbi at the pulpit. As I opened the service with the Blessing of the Sabbath, my strong tenor voice startled the two dozen aging congregants who were present. They looked up in amazement as my voice echoed throughout the synagogue, bringing it to life again. I sang each prayer with a feeling and spirit I had never experienced before. I actually felt part of the ancient tradition of the Jewish community of Pisa.

When the services were over, Rabbi Attilio laid his small bony hand on my shoulder.

"You will be fine, Guido. You have captured the soul of the music. You are a link in our chain. *Ye shar koach,*" he said, which means "blessed be thy strength." Then the rabbi turned to the members of the congregation, who had come up to congratulate me on my first evening as chasan (cantor), and they began to sing the *"Hatikva,"* the song of hope and the Israeli national anthem. Everyone joined in. I felt so proud at that moment!

✳ ✳ ✳

That night Rabbi Attilio died peacefully in his sleep. His wife called me early in the morning and asked me to officiate at the funeral that afternoon. The whole Jewish community was present for the services and mourned the death of their rabbi. For this dwindling community, his death almost seemed to symbolize the end of their whole tradition.

After services, each mourner spent a few moments in silent prayer or thought over Rabbi Attilio's grave and then, gradually, they drifted away. As I turned to leave, a flock of pigeons descended on the freshly dug earth, cooing.

Did they know it was Rabbi Attilio's final resting place? I watched them as they suddenly took flight. All except two: Bubale and Zubale. To this day I believe they knew, and chose to remain close their friend the rabbi. I never saw them any place else again.

XV

Rome and the Two German Shepherds

✳

We remained in Pisa another two years. I continued my duties as *chasan*, though without Rabbi Attilio to teach me, I never progressed beyond the Friday night service! My wife had begun to study singing with *maestro* Picci, a dear man who refused to accept any money for the lessons he gave her. We were still saving about half my monthly allotment, but life was more fun now. My involvement with the synagogue and my wife's singing created many opportunities to expand our circle of friends. Italians have a deep love for music and eagerly embrace those who share their passion. Many of the friendships we developed continue to this day. So I had mixed emotions when I decided to try for a job I had heard about at the Israeli Embassy in Rome. We had grown to love Pisa, but I knew that the last year in school wouldn't necessitate my full-time presence and the possibility of working for the embassy and living in Rome was irresistible.

By sheer luck, I got the job and we were on our way to new adventures in Rome and the world of diplomacy! The Israeli Embassy was located in a white, two-story building in Parioli, an exclusive suburb. It bustled with intense activity; it was a gateway for the flow of information and goods and a center for both overt and covert diplomatic activities.

My basic job was to file documents, both official and secret. It was important, but not very glamorous. I had other duties as well, more exciting but not glamorous either. Civitavecchia, the port near Rome, was a point of origin for shipments of weapons to Israel. This same port was also used by the Arabs and we had to guard the Israeli ships against sabotage. So from time to time I would be assigned to swim around and under the ships in the harbor, looking for bombs which might have been attached to the hulls. The port waters were oily and murky, and there was always the possibility of being blown up. I never discovered any bombs or sabotage, but it was exciting to look anyway!

I was just a minor functionary at the embassy. Because my wife and I spoke Italian, unlike most of the embassy staff, we were invited to many diplomatic receptions. At first, these receptions were fun, but then they became more of a bore. There were always the same faces, the same endless idle chitchat about topics no one really wanted to discuss, with everyone holding forever the obligatory glass of champagne.

On one particular occasion, the combination of the lateness of the hour and the spiciness of the food made me terribly ill. Almost immediately, we had to excuse ourselves to go to the nearest hospital. I felt like I was dying. The admissions staff were not particularly sympathetic; they directed me to a big room which was really nothing more than the city's drunk tank.

"*Il dottore arriverà subito, signore* [the doctor will arrive soon]," they assured me. Three hours later I still had not been seen by a doctor! Finally, since no physician seemed likely to appear, I decided that I would rather die in bed at home. Fortunately, a hot water bottle and a little tender loving care from my wife proved sufficient to cure my ills. I vowed never to eat lunch at night again, but that proved difficult given the Italian approach to dining hours!

My work schedule at the embassy was more than full-time. In addition to working Monday through Friday, I took weekend duty, which ran from six in the evening Friday to eight in the morning on Monday. My per hour wages were low, but the weekend hours significantly boosted my overall take-home pay and we were able to add almost half of the total salary to our savings. I was determined to have enough money by the time we returned to Israel to buy everything we would need to set up housekeeping in more fitting quarters than we had experienced in Italy.

Every two weeks I returned to Pisa for two or three days to continue my studies. I would take the "red eye" train, sleeping all the way and giving the conductor a big tip to wake me at Pisa. I don't think my professors were too happy with my rather unorthodox attendance, but I hadn't missed a day of class in the first four years and I made sure I was present for every exam.

In Rome we sublet a small room with kitchen and bath privileges in a large, but somewhat shabby house in a run-down area near a wealthy quarter of the city. My memories of the neighborhood revolve almost entirely around the baroness and her enormous German shepherd, Max, who lived across the street from us. Three times a day the baroness would come out of her elegant old house, preceded by Max on a gold-plated leash, with his mouth open and his big red tongue hanging out to one side. Max was truly magnificent and always groomed and brushed until his coat gleamed in the sun. He eclipsed the baroness in grandeur, although she was always dressed beautifully, as if she were going to the opera.

I was fascinated by the baroness and Max. First, I had never seen a dog so well groomed; in the Middle East, dogs tend to be unkempt and scroungy. Second, and more importantly, there was something mysterious about their relationship. They were so perfectly in tune as they walked down the street. So sedate. So reserved. I always exchanged nods and perhaps a *"Buona sera* [good evening]" with the baroness as I passed them on my way home. I never dared say more, as neither Max nor the baroness were the sort that invited casual acquaintance or friendly conversation.

I soon learned that the job of keeping Max beautifully groomed fell to Rosina, one of the baroness' maids. I had gotten in the habit of visiting the neighborhood pet store often to talk with other animal lovers. Rosina was a frequent visitor to the store, too, purchasing various articles for Max, and we soon got to know each other.

Once she learned that I was both her neighbor and nearly a veterinarian, she began to ask my opinion on various soaps and other grooming articles. Of course, I didn't really know very much about this sort of thing. But I was always very happy to offer my opinion.

"You certainly spend a lot of time taking care of Max," I commented one day. "I have never seen a dog with a coat so beautiful. You must spend hours brushing him!"

"Oh yes, *signor dottore,*" she said, and of course, I didn't mind this slight exaggeration of my status, "Max must always be perfect for the baroness. After all, he is much more than her dog, as you know." She smiled a mysterious smile and left the store. Much more than her dog? As I knew? I shrugged, thinking she was slightly strange, and turned my attention to other people in the shop.

※ ※ ※

A few months later, on a Sunday afternoon when I happened to be home, I saw Rosina run out of the baroness' house directly across the street toward our house. I opened the door to a breathless Rosina.

"Please come right away, *signor dottore,*" she said. "Max has caught a fishhook in his lip and is bleeding badly. It is terrible. The baroness is in agony watching him suffer. Our veterinarian is hunting in the country. You must help us."

I wasn't sure I could help, as I had no surgical instruments or drugs, but I agreed to take a look at Max. We entered the baroness' elegant home and Rosina led me straight to the boudoir. The baroness was seated on her satin-covered bed, holding Max's head in her lap. He was bleeding profusely and moaning.

"*Dottore,* you must save my only love, my Maxie." There were tears in her eyes. "We went fishing as we do every Sunday. Max always carries the pole. I don't know how it happened but somehow he caught the hook in his lip! You must help!"

"Bring me a cup of wine mixed with grappa, Rosina. Also bring a pair of pliers," I ordered. "Don't worry," I told the baroness, although I wasn't entirely sure that what I had in mind would work.

Rosina returned with a bottle of very expensive wine and a bottle of grappa on a silver tray. We poured equal amounts into a big bowl and gave it to Max who lapped it up despite his condition. Within a very few minutes, he was nicely asleep, and quite drunk. I began removing the fishhook. Fortunately, it wasn't embedded too deeply. By cutting the tip of the hook, I was able to get it out with the pliers and with only minimal damage to Max.

"Oh, thank you, thank you, *dottore,*" cried the baroness when it was over, grabbing my hand and placing a considerable number of Italian bills in my palm. "You were wonderful. Max and I shall always be grateful."

"Of course, you'll have to take him to his regular doctor tomorrow, baroness. I'm sure he'll want to give him something against infection. Would you like me to move him to the floor, another room . . . his dog house, perhaps?"

"Oh no, *dottore,* thank you so much. Max must remain here with me."

Rosina smiled to me that same smile at the door.

"Don't you understand?" Rosina whispered to me as she ushered me out. "Max is like her husband. He sleeps in the bed with her. They love each other!"

I was aghast. This was not something my veterinary textbooks had prepared me for! I had been treating her lover, not her pet!

Word of my service to Max spread through the neighborhood, where apparently everyone but me already knew of the special relationship between the baroness and Max. From then on I became known as the "Veterinarian of Baron Max."

✳ ✳ ✳

Fortunately, or perhaps unfortunately, nothing else so startling or unusual occurred during the rest of our stay in Rome. We spent our scarce free time enjoying the beauty of the city, and especially its opera and music, the beauty of the Vatican and the endless parks and *piazzas.*

Finally the time came for our return to Israel. Despite my relative absence from school during the last year, I graduated slightly ahead of schedule and with honors. Those years of hard work and concentrated effort paid off.

Our frugality paid off, too. Following graduation we took all our savings and bought every possible household appliance you could imagine, plus a car. When I left on the small munitions ship, Ashkelon, for the return trip to Israel, I had thirty-two suitcases and as many boxes and crates! (My wife and little Fafa would come later on a passenger ship.)

The *Ashkelon* was quite unlike the ship which had brought me to Italy. It was an old freighter, rusty both inside and out, and the captain and his crew matched the unkempt state of the ship. Once on board, I immediately made the acquaintance of another German shepherd, Samba, the captain's dog. He must have sensed my love for animals because he became my constant companion during the voyage. He was certainly a contrast to the regal Max. Overweight from eating table scraps, exuberantly friendly, and scroungy, I often wondered what he would have thought of Max and his life.

It was Samba who first sensed our approach to land. His barking woke the ship at sunrise on the fourth day of the voyage. Faintly, on the horizon, I could see my homeland again — for the first time in five years. Tears welled up in my eyes. I was home. Ready to serve my country in the profession I had chosen: Doctor Sorokin. And unlike during my first voyage, this time the doctor title was genuine!

XVI

The Provincial Government Vet

*

I hated my first job as a vet.

The 1956 war with Egypt had just ended when I arrived back in Israel. The country was still recovering, and still in infancy. Because of the severe shortage of veterinarians, I envisioned myself doing clinical work almost immediately, solving complicated veterinary problems, treating mysteriously sick animals, inventing novel and better ways of dealing with traditional diseases: my vision and reality were worlds apart.

In 1956 there were only about five veterinarians in private practice in Israel and I was too "green" a veterinarian to even consider the possibility of setting up my own practice. The only other jobs for veterinarians in the country were controlled by the government and by the Hachaklait Insurance Company, a semi-private veterinary health maintenance organization, or HMO.

I desperately wanted to be a "field" vet, assigned to the Hachaklait. So the day following my return to Israel, I drove to the Hachaklait main office in Haifa.

After a brief wait, I was ushered into the office of Dr. Schturman, the head of medical services. He listened very patiently while I reviewed my education and qualifications and told him of my desire to work with the Hachaklait.

"Dr. Sorokin," he finally interrupted. "We would be delighted to have your services, but unfortunately we have just hired a new veterinarian. As you know there is a terrible shortage of veterinarians here. They are needed for all kinds of jobs, both with us and with the government. Therefore, the government and the Hachaklait have agreed that any new veterinarians coming to Israel will be alternately assigned, one to the government, one to the Hachaklait, one to the government, etc. So, under our agreement with the government, we cannot hire anyone else now until the government has hired someone. You must approach the Department of Agriculture in Jerusalem."

"But I don't want to work for the Department of Agriculture," I exclaimed. "That's a horrible job. No one practices medicine there. They are just a bunch of paper-shufflers!"

Dr. Schturman shook his head slowly, smiling ruefully. "I'm sorry, young man, but you must understand these circumstances. If you want to practice veterinary medicine in Israel, you'll have to go along with it."

Deeply disappointed, I got back in my car and headed for the Judean Hills in Jerusalem. During the drive I resolved not to just "go along with it." "This is crazy!" I thought. "This country is desperate for veterinarians. There must be a way around this ridiculous gentleman's agreement." By the time I arrived in Jerusalem, I was convinced of it.

But convincing Drs. Gur and Freund, heads of Veterinary Services of the Department of Agriculture, was another matter. "You are, of course, entitled to your views about the nature of veterinary practice offered by the government in contrast to that offered by the Hachaklait," they responded coolly, following my impassioned dissertation on the subject.

They smiled and shrugged in the face of my youthful arrogance and straightforward declaration, "I don't want to work for you!" Worse yet, they were unwilling to discuss any revisions to the rule. "There are no exceptions, Dr. Sorokin." Each time I tried to suggest an alternative arrangement, they would simply shake their heads and reiterate, "But, that is not how things are, young man. If you want to practice veterinary medicine in Israel, you will have to go along."

"This is slavery!" I argued. "You are forcing me to leave the country!"

"No, no. Of course not," said Dr. Freund in a soothing voice. "But, if you want to practice veterinary medicine in Israel, you'll have to. . . ."

"I'm sick of that phrase and I won't go along!" I interrupted, shouting, "even if I have to leave the country!" I stormed out of the office and drove back home to Ramatayim.

I have to admit, I pouted in Ramatayim for over two weeks. Of course, at that time I considered myself "on strike" rather than sulking. During the two weeks, I railed on, to anyone who would listen, about the stupid government and Hachaklait bureaucracy. I threatened to publicly challenge their agreement as an illegal labor practice. I schemed about returning to Italy to work with one of my favorite professors at the university. I dreamt about starting my own practice. And finally, I realized that none of my grandiose schemes were very sensible and that I'd better try to work things out with the government.

I returned to Jerusalem in a more rational and conciliatory mood with a proposal that I accept the Department of Agriculture job for a period of one year, after which I would be free to go to work for the Hachaklait. Somewhat to my surprise, Dr. Freund agreed to this compromise, and even agreed to assign me to the Department of Agriculture's brand new Office of Veterinary Services, which was just being established in the province of Ashkelon. I have always suspected that his acceptance of this compromise was more enlightened self-interest than a true change of heart. Israel is a very small country and my threats to publicly challenge the "gentleman's agreement" had probably reached his ears, even in Jerusalem. Possible scandal was certainly to be avoided. The government had enough problems as it was! Whatever the reason, however, I was pleased with the proposed assignment.

Ashkelon is a very old city built largely on sand dunes in the southern region of Israel, just north of the Gaza Strip. It was one of five ancient Philistine cities, later flourishing under the Romans and gradually decaying. In more modern times it had housed a small Arab population until the War of Independence, when it was largely abandoned. The city was resettled by Jews following the war. While the old part of the city remained much as it had been before the war, new quarters had been established largely with donations from South African Jews. The growth of the surrounding province was made possible by the water carrier built in the early years of the State of Israel to bring water from the river Yarkon. With water available, cattle raising and agriculture became possible allowing the town to grow.

The Department of Agriculture's Office of Veterinary Services in Ashkelon was located in a new, prefabricated building in downtown Ashkelon. The office was Spartan and not much to talk about, but I was thrilled with the new pick-up truck I was given to use in carrying out my duties throughout the province.

I was to be the only government vet for the province, but I was allowed to hire a veterinary assistant. After interviewing a number of candidates, none of whom knew very much, if anything, about veterinary medicine, I chose Izzi. He was known to be a pretty good worker, but I chose him mainly because he was Italian. After only a few weeks back in Israel, I was "homesick" for Italy and the carefree spirit of the Italians. I hoped Izzi would help alleviate some of the tedium I knew was coming with this job!

The work of the provincial office was mainly regulatory, concentrating on the prevention of infectious diseases through testing and inoculation. I thought this was about as boring a job as could be imagined and voiced my views at every opportunity.

My supervisor was Dr. Shoshan, an older man who had been in government veterinary services all his life, originally during the British Mandate and then under the Israeli Government. His passion was the history of veterinary medicine, particularly in the Middle East. He was personally dedicated to understanding and rationalizing ancient commands and events in the Bible and Koran in accordance with contemporary veterinary medical knowledge.

Dr. Shoshan viewed his job with the government almost as a sacred mission and he couldn't understand why I found it boring.

"Your comments belittle the importance of our profession, Doctor!" He finally exploded on my second day of training. "Don't you understand that humanity's attempt to eradicate disease in animals has a very ancient history? Our own dietary laws originated from painstaking observation of the effect of animal diseases on man. Early attempts at disease eradication even appear in the Bible. You know the story of Jesus and the swine? According to the story, Jesus cast out devils from tormented souls and sent the devils into a herd of swine. The swine went mad and ran headlong down a steep hill into the Sea of Galilee where they were drowned.

"Now in Tabcha, the area in which this 'miracle' took place, pigs have long been infested with leptospirosis, even to this day, which you know causes a behavior akin to madness and is ultimately fatal in both pigs and man. Don't you see that the 'devils' that caused this madness in the Biblical story are a reflection of the people's experience with the disease. You might say Jesus helped foster efforts to eradicate it! The same job we have, Doctor! You should be proud of your work. It is critical to saving lives. Sure, there's paperwork, sure there's repetitive tasks, but think of the results we are trying to achieve."

I was a bit surprised by the comparison to Jesus, but the good doctor's words and his personal dedication were not lost on me. I began to look at the work differently, with a greater sense of importance and pride in the task I had been assigned.

My first assignment was tuberculin testing of all the cows in the province. Now, you will recall that my Italian education was strong on theory and very short on practical experience! In short, I was about as "green" a doctor as you can get and my tuberculin testing duties were the first real "hands-on" clinical experience I had ever had.

The farmers in the province used to tease me that they could always tell a new vet "by the smell." In my case, it was regrettably true, at least for the first few weeks as I learned to work with the animals. Each day I would start out spic and span and each night I would return covered with dirt and cow manure.

The tuberculin testing involved shaving two square patches on the side of the cow's neck, cleansing the skin with alcohol, and carefully injecting one patch intradermally with a tenth of a centigram of bovine tuberculosis and the other with a tenth of a centigram of chicken tuberculosis. The cows were in individual, narrow stalls. I would enter the stall from the rear and attempt to maneuver around the cow to begin preparations for the injection while the farmer or a hired hand held the cow's nose with a special nose gripper.

My patients were not patient with me! They reacted to my inexpert advances with every weapon they had: horns, teeth, legs, tails and projectile squirts from their hind quarters! I was black and blue from being stepped on, bumped and even knocked to the floor. At least once a day during those first few weeks one of the cows would score a direct hit of some sort or other, unfortunately usually of the odorific kind. It was many weeks before I learned to relate to the animals and to anticipate their sudden moves and tricks.

The farmers and their hired hands were always amused with my struggles. A few of them even tried some tricks of their own.

"My best cow has lost all her upper teeth, Doc," said Isaac to me one day in a serious tone in the presence of a number of his workers. "Do you Italian vets know anything about bovine dentistry?" Isaac was a wizened old farmer who had raised cows for years and probably knew more about their care and treatment than most vets. Of course, I knew that cows have no teeth on their upper front jaw and was really annoyed that Isaac thought he might be able to fool me with such a stupid comment.

"Sorry, Isaac, my specialty is elephant tusks and crooked alligator teeth. Looks like you yourself could use my services, judging from those crooked yellow fangs you've got! If you like I will throw in a hair transplant for your shiny head, too. Your brains must be escaping through your bald spot if you think you could trick me with such nonsense about cow teeth!"

Isaac laughed, but I noticed he covered his mouth with his hands to hide his perfectly awful teeth.

Gaining the respect of the farmers was a tough proposition for a greenhorn vet for a more serious reason. When a tuberculin test showed positive, the farmer was required to send the cow to the slaughterhouse and generally would receive inadequate compensation from the government for the animal. Positive test results were not well received! There was always a challenge, even when the results were obvious. "You must have done the test wrong. Don't you know a false positive when you see one, greenhorn? This is my best cow. I'm not taking her anywhere until an experienced vet sees her!" Since the vast majority of farmers actually watched all tuberculin testing of their herds and knew perfectly well the difference between a positive and a false positive result, I gradually realized their comments were largely a result of frustration rather than any serious questioning of my skill. But their carrying on was hard on my ego, and once or twice led me to doubt myself.

One such instance of doubt arose after I finished testing a herd in Kfar Warburg. The owner, Mrs. Cohen, had not been present when I did the testing, which I had erroneously taken as a sign that she trusted my skill implicitly. Her senior hired hand called me in a panic the morning of the day I was to check the test results.

"Dr. Sorokin, something went really wrong with the testing here. Half the herd looks like positive. You'd better get out here and try it again."

When I arrived at the farm, to my amazement I found that over 50 percent of the herd had reacted positively to the test. This was the largest percentage I had ever seen. I was certain I had done the testing correctly, but I still couldn't believe my eyes. I called my supervisor immediately for consolation just to make sure he agreed with my view that tuberculosis was endemic and had spread to the majority of cows in the Cohen's herd. He came quickly and confirmed the diagnosis.

"Where is Mrs. Cohen?" I asked. "I must let her know right away that the majority of the herd will have to be destroyed." I knew this would be economic disaster and dreaded having to tell her.

"Oh, you can't tell her this now," exclaimed the dairy supervisor. "She's very sick. She's been in the hospital a number of days now, Doctor. Some mysterious disease which she got from her husband. He died from it! And we are really worried about her. The doctors can't seem to diagnose it. You must not disturb her!"

Dr. Shoshan and I exchanged glances. I immediately went to the phone and called the local hospital and Mrs. Cohen's doctor.

"Try testing Mrs. Cohen for bovine tuberculosis, Doctor. I will bet you'll solve your diagnosis problem."

I was right! Mrs. Cohen's cows went to slaughter, but she recuperated quickly following treatment with the proper antibiotics. I felt tremendous professional pride in having contributed to saving her life.

Another of my jobs as a provincial government vet was working to eradicate rabies. This was a noble aim, critical to saving human as well as animal lives. The process, however was horrible and provided me with my first real experience with truly distasteful veterinary work.

Following the 1956 war, rabies had become a particularly serious problem in Israel. The valleys in southern Israel were strewn with the leftovers of battle consisting not only of abandoned and disabled vehicles and weapons, but also of the dead and decomposing bodies of Egyptian soldiers which had yet to be removed or buried. Hyenas, jackals, dogs and vultures congregated to feast on the grisly results of battle. The population of animals of prey multiplied, and with it the incidence of rabies.

To combat the problem, the government issued an order to poison all stray dogs and wild animals. My job was to travel throughout the valleys and desert areas of the province depositing rations laced with strychnine, "land mines," so to speak, in the war against rabies. My assistant Izzi and I would return three days later to collect the uneaten bait. We would find hundreds of dead and bloated bodies of the animals that had eaten the poisoned flesh of those who had died from the poison. It was a terrible sight and the stench was sickening. The method was crude, but at that time it was considered essential to protect the human population against potentially horrible death from rabies. The job made my resolve to leave government service at the end of the year even stronger.

Socially, my family and I were very happy in Ashkelon. The government had helped us get a loan to buy half of a new duplex in Afridar, the part of Ashkelon which had been created with money donated by South African Jews. Our neighbors were from all over the world: Germany, South Africa, Poland, Italy, Romania, Hungary, even India — a microcosm of the immigrant population in Israel. Most were middle class and many of them worked in the local factory which made the big pipes for the national water carrier. In our neighborhood there were a few professionals among us, two other veterinarians who worked for the Hachaklait, one physician, and one lawyer.

Yoram Golan, the lawyer, was passionately interested in arts and music and all things cultural. Together we founded a social club to promote cultural activities, lectures, concerts, and to integrate all the cultures brought to Israel by the immigrants. My wife frequently entertained with her singing and I used to lecture about life in Italy, veterinary medicine, and anything else I could get an audience to listen to. Yoram used to entertain us with jokes and our Indian neighbors taught us to appreciate Indian music. Despite all our different backgrounds, the social club helped create a sense of community among us.

Ashkelon, like most of Israel, was governed by a socialist coalition.

As in most towns, the head of the trade union, the Histadrut, was the local political "king-maker." In Ashkelon this person was Yaacov. Like all his counterparts throughout Israel, Yaacov took his orders from the head of the union in Tel Aviv. The strength of the Histradrut was such that the headquarters in Tel Aviv were jokingly nicknamed the "Kremlin." Whatever the Kremlin ordered was spread throughout Israel through the local unions.

In those days I was a borderline Socialist, generally voting with the Labor Party, although concerned with the socialist regime's undue restriction of enterprise and competition. For example, the inefficiencies and poor quality control of the local water-pipe factory, which was mostly government owned, were well known throughout the community. Given the importance of the water carrier factory, its operation was a topic of intense discussion and debate, and I was never one to shy away from such a chance!

"You won't believe it, Yehudale [I had resumed my Israeli name when I returned from Italy]," said my Indian neighbor one day when we met at the social club. He was a welder at the factory.

"I worked my tail off today. We have a major job to finish for the expansion of the water carrier and at least three of the most important workers just sit around and do nothing all day. They know they will get paid even if they don't work. So they decide not to bother when it gets too hot! It's really disgusting!"

By this time Yaacov had joined us. "What do you say, Yaacov? How will we ever complete the pipeline construction for the connection to the Lake Kineret portion of the water project if half your workers sleep on the job?" I exaggerated with a smile just to get the conversation going as a small crowd gathered.

"When you cut wood, there are always a lot of splinters!" he replied. "Let's look at the great achievements, the wondrous things that the workers have accomplished. Not this piddling stuff. These complaints are nothing when you think of what we have created with this water carrier and this factory. Together they will revolutionize Israel, making agriculture possible where it has never been before!"

"True," I replied, "but that doesn't mean you should not tighten up the controls and efficiency of the factory, Yaacov. Think how much more we would accomplish if everyone would give one hundred percent instead of just waiting around for his paycheck! I think my Indian friend is only interested in helping to bring about your dream, everyone's dream, a little faster!"

"Say, Yehuda, what are you doing? Running for office?" someone in the crowd called out "You are sounding every day more and more like a politician making speeches!"

"Not me," I laughed. "The combination of government bureaucracy, trade union control, and all these crazy Jews from all over the world with different ideas about how things should be run . . . why, it would drive me crazy!"

Through my participation in the social club and in political discussions (which in Ashkelon were almost constant) and through my veterinary travels around the province, I quickly became well known throughout both town and countryside. As the months passed, I gradually gained the professional respect of the farmers I dealt with and even began to develop personal friendships with a number of them. Little by little they would start to ask me to perform veterinary services that weren't strictly within my role as a provincial government vet. I was flattered and also excited by these opportunities to practice "real" veterinary medicine.

Now you may think from my comments that "real" veterinary medicine was more glamorous than the sorts of projects I had as a government vet. But there was no glamor in my first "real" job.

I had scheduled a vaccination against anthrax and blue tongue for the flock of Mr. Elias, the town pharmacist and practically the last Arab in Ashkelon. He watched the whole process from his porch, smoking his *narghile* (water pipe), dressed in the traditional white robes, with his head covered by his spotless white kafia held in place by a black *agal*.

Elias was a Christian with a great deal of property in the Ashkelon area. In contrast to the majority of Arabs who lived in Ashkelon prior to 1948, Elias did not flee to Jordan after the War of Independence. Unlike his brethren, he had faith in the assurances of his Jewish friends in the area that he would be treated fairly. And he had been. He was accepted and respected in the community. Nonetheless, he kept himself apart and even sent his children overseas to study. His obvious minority position in the town in which he was raised and which used to be 100 percent Arab, must have been difficult for him to accept psychologically.

After the vaccination job was completed, he called me over to the house and offered me, as is customary, Turkish coffee and *baklava* (a sweet Turkish pastry). The conversation proceeded in the traditional manner, polite inquiries about each other's families and work, a little discussion about local politics, appropriate expressions of appreciation for the government's free vaccination program and the fact that his farm was serviced with the rest of the farmers of the province. At the end, he turned to me and said, "Say, I know it's not your job, Doc, but would you mind taking a look at one of my rams? He's being eaten alive by an infestation of maggots underneath his tail. I don't know what to do, and there are no private veterinarians in this part of the country."

We walked over to the barn and I checked over the ram, which was lying listlessly on his side and was indeed suffering from a very bad infestation. The area underneath a sheep's tail is warm and moist. When the wool becomes matted, the moisture can't escape and it becomes a perfect incubator for the eggs of flies, as it had in this case. When the eggs hatch, the maggots begin to feed on the flesh of the sheep.

"Can you do anything, Doc?" he asked. "I'm afraid I'm going to lose this one. . . ."

"Well, we'll see," I said. "I can only try. I will have to dig out the maggots one by one. It may take some time." There were big holes in the flesh and hundreds of maggots. Despite the smell and the heat, I set to work with vigor. This was the type of medicine I was meant to practice. Helping sick animals recover. One by one I pulled out the maggots with tweezers and put them in a bucket of water to drown.

While I was engaged in this work, out of nowhere appeared Yaacov. "I've been looking for you everywhere, Doc. What are you doing? It looks pretty disgusting! What kind of work is that for an important doctor like you? Pulling maggots from a sheep's rear in the burning sun!"

I was not allowed to get a word in edgewise. Yaacov went on. "We've got big plans for you, Doc. The Labor Party wants you to run as our candidate for mayor! You've got name recognition throughout the province. The farmers love you, the townspeople know you from the social club. You're not afraid to say what you think, but you are a good socialist, like your Papa. Its a shoo-in, Yehuda. What do you think? It's an offer of a lifetime. You can't refuse!"

I was stunned and tempted at the same time, although in my view politicians ranked only slightly ahead of maggots in the scheme of the universe.

I looked down at the ram, still suffering in the heat. He turned his head to look at me, as if to say, "Please help." I turned back to Yaacov. "I am deeply honored, Yaacov. But I really would make a terrible politician. This is the work I was meant to do. My heart is here, not in politics."

"You prefer to take care of maggots rather than to become mayor?" he asked incredulously. "You must be crazy! I tell you, this is a chance of a lifetime!" But, seeing that I was not to be persuaded, he jumped back in his dusty jeep and drove off, still in a huff that I had refused his remarkable offer.

I finished my job with the ram, shaving the affected area and cleansing it with a disinfectant, then injecting the sheep with antibiotics. The ram was still very weak and sick, but I was certain he would be all right and told Elias so.

"I cannot tell you how grateful I am, Doc," said Elias after I had finished and had explained to him how to help protect his animals from such problems in the future. A a token of his gratitude, he gave me a big circle of home made cheese. I was tired but very happy. From that moment I knew that I had chosen the right profession, even if I had to wait a few more months to complete my year with the government in order to begin the work I loved.

Actually, the remainder of the year went by very quickly, and almost without any major incident. However, shortly before the end of the year, Izzi and I had to vaccinate a herd of Brahma cattle. Izzi didn't always accompany me on these vaccination visits, but Brahma are so dangerous that I knew I would need his help in addition to the help of the cowboys.

"You know these cows don't speak Italian, Izzi," I said jokingly to him. He was a great one for trying to "sweet talk" the animals. "I wouldn't try your usual tactics. If you get as close as you usually do, you will end up with a horn in your face!"

We drove about an hour into the semi-desert area where the herd had been rounded up. There were several hundred head of the hump-backed, big horned animals pacing nervously in the makeshift corral.

The cowboys began the work of singling out the cattle, pushing them one by one into a chute. They would run pell-mell to the end, pushing to get out. At the end of the chute was a head-high opening. The cattle would push their heads into the opening and a triangular bar would fall into place, trapping the head. Izzi and I stood along side and when the animal was trapped, I injected the vaccine. Izzi kept me supplied with filled syringes as the animals raced through the chute. There was no time to waste as the animals were quite violent and capable of breaking the chute down.

Finally, there was only one steer left, but he was not about to enter the chute. He paced the corral, evading the cowboys by picking up speed whenever they got close. Three of the cowboys, mounted on horses, began to circle the bull and edge him towards the chute. Just as he was about to enter, he turned his head viciously and gored the horse on his left. The horse neighed in pain, lost its balance, and fell. Somehow the rider ended up under the horse. In the commotion, the bull turned back and ran into the shoot. He was frothing at the mouth and obviously terrified. It was pandemonium; we were all scared. Somehow I managed to vaccinate him and get him out of the chute before he broke it down with his wild thrashing. Then I quickly jumped over the fence into the corral to help the horse and rider. The cowboy had a severely broken leg and pelvis and I couldn't really do anything for him except help load him on the truck and take him to the hospital.

I turned my attention to the horse. The wound was bleeding profusely, but it wasn't really as bad as it first appeared. I dressed the wound, injected the horse with antibiotics, and told the cowboys to call the Hachaklait vets as soon as possible. I was exhausted. It was one of the most violent occurrences I ever experienced in my veterinary career.

Finally, after several more vaccination projects and several extremely boring ear-tagging identification projects, my year in government service drew to a close. My replacement was a fat Polish immigrant who loved paper work and administration. He was perfectly suited for the job.

"We will miss you, Dr. Sorokin," said Dr. Shoshan. "You brought a lot of spirit and energy to your work, even if we never convinced you of its importance."

"I appreciate all the help you have given me, Dr. Shoshan," I replied. "Although you didn't make a government vet out of me, you were very supportive and a good man to work for!"

I collected my gear from the office and left without regret to begin my career with the Hachaklait.

XVII

Cows, Cows, Cows

*

I kissed my wife with great fervor, patted sleeping Fafa on the head, grabbed my suitcase, and jumped into my old Opel car. The motor sprang to life and I roared down the street. This was the day I had been waiting for. I was finally going to work for the Hachaklait, the animal HMO of Israel responsible for actual treatment of most farm animals in the country.

The sun was just peaking over the Judean hills as I headed out of Ashkelon for Haifa, where the Hachaklait's main office was located. I recalled my first visit there after my return from Italy, my disappointment, my anger at not being allowed to work there. "Well, this will be different," I thought to myself. "I have paid my dues to the government and done a damn good job as a provincial vet. I have proven myself a hard worker and a man who can be trusted. Now let's see how this interview goes!" As I sped along the road to Haifa I imagined Dr. Schturman greeting me warmly. "Well, you've finally made it, Doctor Sorokin! We have been waiting and watching your progress. We are really pleased to have a veterinarian of your caliber so anxious to join us!"

Fortunately, there were no police on the road that morning. My speed increased as my imaginary conversations grew more and more elaborate and complimentary. By the time I pulled into the driveway at the Hachaklait, my heart was pounding a mile a minute. I forced myself to sit a minute in the car after I parked, trying to calm down so I would present just the right professional image at the interview.

As I approached the main entrance to the building, the familiar, almost overwhelming, odor of drugs burst into my face from the pharmacy window on the right: a blend of sweet molasses, camphor, ether and other chemicals. From the corner of my eye, I saw a bald head and an old, wrinkled face peaking out of the second story window. Dr. Schturman, the head veterinarian of the Hachaklait! My heart started pounding again as I climbed the stairs to his office. He strode out of his office to meet me, tall and slender, his bald head gleaming under the fluorescent lights and his white lab coat hanging open over his street clothes.

"So, Dr. Sorokin, the famous *dottore italiano* that always gets his way with government bureaucracy! Welcome back!"

"Thank you very much, Dr. Schturman," I responded enthusiastically. "You know how much I want to be here!"

"We're all impressed with your determination," he responded drily, his cigarette dangling carelessly from his mouth. "But, you know we have our own form of bureacracy at the Hachaklait. What makes you think you'll be able to manage here, my young *dottore italiano?*" he asked with a smile that revealed his tobacco-stained teeth.

"Well, to work for the Hachaklait is my dream," I responded. "To really treat animals, help relieve their suffering. This is the work I really want to do. You'll see. I'll work incredibly hard for you."

Dr. Schturman interrupted, turning to lead me into the main office. "This is the place for hard work, all right! I'm sure you'll be fine as long as you remember to play by the rules!" He turned and raised his eyebrows at me questioningly.

"Of course, of course," I responded quickly, not really understanding what he meant. I was too excited to be concerned about whether or not the Hachaklait was as bureaucratic as the government. Only much later was I to appreciate the significance of this early "play by the rules" admonition.

The office was enormous and incredibly cluttered. Dr. Schturman's huge desk was at one end, piled high with files and medicine bottles. There were books and magazines from all over the world in stacks on every table and on many of the chairs. There were even piles of papers and books on the floor. At the opposite end of the room, seated in the corner in a big over-stuffed chair that had seen better days, behind an absolutely immaculate and clear glass-topped desk, was a serious-looking, slightly pudgy man, with heavy horn-rimmed glasses. His face gave the impression of a studious rabbi, but he had no beard and was dressed in a khaki shirt and pants and work boots like a farmer.

"This is Avram Joffe, our Chief Executive Officer," Dr. Schturman explained.

Mr. Joffe rose to shake my hand. "Dr. Sorokin, we've heard mostly good things about you. You seem to be a hard worker. You have to understand," he said sternly, "this is not an eight-hour a day job. There is very little paper shuffling here! It's blood, sweat, and frustration. And, you'll have to please every farmer. Each one will think he is your boss because he pays ten pounds a year for his insurance premium!

"Keeping the farmers happy is every bit as important as working with the animals. We've got a business to run. From what I hear, you are a pretty outspoken young man. Can you learn to keep your mouth shut when necessary?"

I squirmed a little and felt my face grow hot. Diplomacy was not my forte and no one had ever quite so bluntly told me I would have to play politics to be a successful Hachaklait veterinarian. The interview was not progressing in the manner I had envisioned in the car earlier that morning!

Dr. Schturman took over. "We've had quite a few interesting experiences with you 'spaghetti vets,' you know. You're all great on theory, but some of you don't even know from which end a cow pees! Of course, you have all got a line of bull that helps hide your lack of practical experience."

I laughed uneasily, wishing the interview would end and wondering what this was all leading to.

"You have to admit there have been a few great Italians," I responded starting to name a few. "Leonardo da Vinci, Enrico Fermi, . . ."

Mr. Joffe cut me off with a look and Dr. Schturman rejoined, "So far none of them veterinarians who have returned to practice in Israel! Anyway, that is not the point. As you know, all our new vets go through a one month internship. In your case, because of your lack of practical experience, we have decided to assign you to Dr. Sirron. This will be an intense experience. Dr. Sirron is not only an excellent veterinarian, he is one of our hardest workers. And tough! He will not make it any easier for you just because you come to us barely knowing which end of a cow is which!" he laughed.

"Yes, you'll have to behave yourself with Dr. Sirron. And with his wife Lina. She's the real boss in the family." He winked at me and shook his head. I heard him mutter to himself quietly,

`"Poor Dr. Sirron!"

The business part of the interview ended. Dr. Schturman's assistant brought in cups of steaming tea and Turkish coffee and the atmosphere subtly changed. They no longer treated me like an inexperienced school kid. The conversation turned to Israeli politics. The previous evening there had been another *fedayin* (guerrillas) infiltration from the Gaza Strip. The infiltrators had attacked a kibbutz, but had not managed to kill anybody this time.

"I think we should get licenses for our vets working in security zones to carry Sten guns [predecessors of Uzis]," said Joffe. "The situation is getting serious and the chances of the government getting things under control soon are slim."

"You may be right," responded Schturman, "but we are really talking mostly about psychological value. After all, if someone waits for you on the highway at night, there isn't much you can do to protect yourself. But it might be worth considering."

"You know it's not only the *fedayin* our vets have to worry about, Dr. Sorokin." said Joffe. "These ultra-religious types are making things more and more difficult now. Why, only last week Dr. Shomron was stoned by a group of zealots as he was rushing to the aid of a horse on Yom Kippur. The horse would have died if the doctor had not arrived when he did, and those fools actually stoned him and tried to prevent him from doing his job! Do they think the horse knew it was Yom Kippur? And, of course, we would have had to pay the farmer for the dead horse if they had succeeded. Imagine!" He shook his head. I wasn't sure whether he was more concerned about saving the horse or the insurance payment.

"Of course, the job is not really all that dangerous," Dr. Schturman hastened to add. He must have sensed that I was getting a little nervous. "We don't want you to think you will always have to live in fear for your life. There are many benefits to consider. We pay for your car and your residence. And, if you do the job right, everyone will look up to you. You might even get asked to run for mayor! We have a couple of vets who now have that honor in their home towns."

"Well, I think I've lost my chance for that, Dr. Schturman," I replied, recounting the story of my preference for maggots over politicians in Ashkelon.

Mr. Joffe and Dr. Schturman laughed. "Probably a wise choice," they said. "Besides you'll have your hands full working for us now! For new vets there's no time for extracurricular politics!"

Finally Dr. Schturman arose. "Well, Doctor, you'd better be getting along to Dr. Sirron's house. You will stay with him at his home for the entire month. After his report to us on your progress, we shall see where your first real assignment will be."

* * *

Dr. Sirron lived about a half an hour drive from Haifa on the way to Nazareth. The area is hilly, green and wooded, different from the typical arid sand dunes and mountains of the Israeli landscape. As I drove, I tried to remember everything I had heard about Dr. Sirron, who was second in command of the professional veterinary services of the Hachaklait, directly under Dr. Schturman. I had never seen him, but I'd been told he looked like a big bear, hairy all over except for his scalp, which was completely bald. Dr. Sirron had come to Israel from Lithuania, and shared many of the characteristics of Jewish Lithuanians: he was serious, knowledgeable, studious, hard-working and fair. Dr. Sirron was said to be extremely stern, and people feared him more than Dr. Schturman, who was known to have a big bark but very little bite. Oddly, at home, Dr. Sirron was supposedly under the complete domination of his wife, Lina.

Lina and her relationship with her husband were the source of constant gossip among company veterinarians. I had heard that she was extremely good-looking for her age; there were rumors that she had undergone a very expensive face lifting in Paris. Rumors also alleged that she was more than friendly with her husband's trainees. I must admit, I was curious about meeting her.

I turned into the drive of the Sirron's house. The yard was lovely, a fantastic garden with beautiful flowers and shrubs, all neatly manicured. Lina evidently heard the car drive up, and met me at the door. The stories about her were true. She was indeed good-looking, and dressed extremely well, as if she had just returned from a fancy luncheon. Her blond hair looked freshly done.

She greeted me warmly. "Dr. Sorokin, welcome to your home for the next month. Let me show you to your room and explain the home regulations to you. My husband will keep you busy night and day, but you will also have a few duties around the house in exchange for your room and board." Was it my imagination, or did she wink at me as she said that?

"Don't worry. You won't have to do the dishes or clean up in the kitchen. My husband thinks that these are his sacred duties. Of course, that's about all he does around here — if you know what I mean." Another wink? "Your job will be to keep the garden in perfect order and walk the dogs, Fifi and Tuzzy, twice a day and groom them at night. I hear you studied in Italy. I hope you are not one of these Italian lover boys who only like to sleep, play and make love!" She brushed up against my sleeve, and this time I know there really was another wink. Just then, Lina's daughter Debbie, a plump, unattractive kid appeared.

"Debbie, take Dr. Sorokin to see the shower in the garage." Turning to me she explained, "I can't stand the animal stink you vets come home with. I made Naftali build a shower in the garage so he could clean up before coming into the house. Don't you dare come into the house after work before using that shower!"

Debbie skipped ahead of me to the garage. "Is it true that Italian men are the best lovers?" she asked.

"Well, I wouldn't know, Debbie. I am an Israeli."

"But, you went to school there, didn't you?"

"Yes, but I still don't know the answer to your question."

Fortunately, she seemed to lose interest in the topic and our conversation turned to safer subjects such as her school work, her friends, her pets, her ambitions. "I really want to be a vet like my dad," she said, as we entered the house.

"Good grief, child," said Lina. "Do you want to end up with hair that smells like cow dung and fingernails covered with dirt? Think about a more lady-like career, please." It was obvious that Lina was not particularly supportive of her husband's work and made no bones about it!

About that time we heard the shower water running in the garage. "Well, he's returned early to meet you! Don't get the idea that you'll be home this early every night." Lina laughed harshly.

A few moments later my mentor entered, wearing a bathrobe as if ready for bed after a long day's work. He did look somewhat like a bear, except for his red nose which stuck out prominently. He motioned me to sit at the table while Lina and Debbie prepared dinner.

"So you are the famous Dr. Sorokin that accused the Department of Agriculture of slave trading in veterinarians because you were forced to work there against your will?" He peered intently at me through his thick black glasses. "You are the only one I know who's had the guts to really take on the government. What's more you even had a partial victory!"

"Well," I responded proudly, "I'm a descendant of the Khazars. You know what tough people they were. I guess that toughness is still in my blood."

"Ah, you have a sense of history. Interesting. History is my second love, after veterinary medicine. I am a Lithuanian. Love of learning and love of animals were instilled in me since I was a child. I love my job because it gives me the opportunity to use some of the knowledge I have acquired over the years to help save animals. I'm a simple man, with simple needs. I don't need anything more than a good day's work to make me happy!"

He must have noticed me looking at the fine china and elegant table setting which were in strong contrast to his statement of "simple needs."

"Oh, that . . . that's all Lina's doing," he shrugged. "She is crazy about these things and the house and the yard. She likes to show off to all the wives of the other vets. She thinks I'm crazy for working so hard, but she doesn't mind the things she's able to buy as a result!"

Lina and Debbie entered with the dinner. I was ravenous and really enjoyed the spaghetti and meat sauce she served "in honor of the Italian vet." Dr. Sirron, in contrast, had his mind still on work and on my training which was to begin the next morning.

"For the next month you are going to devote your life to one question: Is the cow pregnant or not, and if she is not, how can we make her pregnant? That's the centerpiece of our work." He lifted his muscular arm and hand straight out over the table and demonstrated, while the rest of us were devouring the spaghetti, "You push your arm up into the cow all the way until you find her ovaries, which are like two small chicken eggs. If the cow is pregnant, at least one of them has to have a particular bulge. That's the *corpus luteum!*"

"Oh I know all about it from our OB/GYN book," I interjected.

Before Sirron could counter with a remark about my lack of practical experience, Debbie jumped in. "Ooh, what does it feel like to push your hand inside a cow?" she inquired, her inquisitive eyes wide open.

"Why, it's warm and squishy. Quite pleasurable, actually, especially on a cold winter day," responded Dr. Sirron to his daughter.

"This is disgusting," exclaimed Lina. "Talking about pushing your arm up cow behinds all day. At dinner! Really, Naftali`. What will Dr. Sorokin think? And what kind of example are you setting for your daughter? How will she ever learn how to hold polite conversation like proper people do?

"Perhaps you are right, dear," answered Dr. Sirron meekly. "Dr. Sorokin and I will continue our conversation in the study after I finish the dishes."

I really liked Dr.Sirron and felt a little sorry for him. Lina was certainly good looking, but she sure made life difficult for him. I was glad I didn't have to put up with her.

"On second thought," said Dr. Sirron. "Let's continue the conversation tomorrow. I will be meeting with the CEO tomorrow before breakfast and want to get a good night's sleep tonight. By the way, you can sleep in, if you want. Enjoy it. It will be the last late morning for the next month!"

I slept like a baby in my fancy room, dreaming that I would soon be able to afford as fine a house for my family as this one. I was awakened by a soft knock at the door just as dawn was breaking.

"Doctor Sorokin, are you still asleep?" It was Lina!

"Just waking," I called. "Am I late?" I asked still sleepy and confused about the time.

"No, no," she responded. "I have your breakfast here." The door swung open and she entered carrying a typical Israeli breakfast on a tray: fresh salad, fish, yogurt, eggs and Turkish coffee. I looked at her in alarm as she entered. She was still in her night clothes and looking quite provocative and more friendly than even I anticipated.

"Did you sleep well, *Bubale*," she asked bending over the bed solicitously and making certain I had an excellent view. This was a dangerous game she wanted to play and I didn't know the rules! If her intentions were as I suspected, and I turned her down, would she hold it against me and take it out on me some way? On the other hand, if her intentions were not as I suspected and I somehow appeared interested, would she hold that against me? Was this some kind of a test to see how I would behave? How was I supposed to behave?

I quickly decided there was too much at stake to do anything other than play this very straight and very innocent. "Breakfast in bed! How extraordinary. My wife," I said with considerable emphasis on the word "wife," "often brings me breakfast in bed. But you really shouldn't Mrs. Sirron. I will join you and your husband in the kitchen. Won't Dr. Sirron be home shortly?" I asked innocently. "I am anxious to get started with my internship. There is so much to learn! I really want to be a good vet. Your husband is supposed to be the best and toughest trainer in the company."

"God deliver me from dedicated veterinarians. They can't get their minds off cows for anything!" Lina said with disgust. "Isn't it enough that I have Naftali to put up with. Now they send trainees who are just like him! You may have gone to school in Italy, but you obviously didn't learn anything useful there!" She put down the tray and swished out of the room.

I sat in stunned silence after she left, wondering what I had gotten myself into in this household. Fortunately, Dr. Sirron returned almost immediately from his early morning meeting, proving that my decision was right not only ethically but also practically!

"Let's go, Dr. Sorokin!" he shouted from the yard. "When I said you could sleep late, I didn't mean all morning!"

I got up quickly, dressed and ran down to the yard where Dr. Sirron was loading his car with needed supplies for the day: antibiotics, syringes and needles, and lots of arm-length gloves for rectal examinations. "Here, put these on," he said tossing me a pair of enormous, heavy coveralls.

"Listen, let me explain our day for you. First we go to Kfar Chasidim, a village of very religious people. They almost won't let in anyone not wearing a hat or *yarmulke*. Of course, they make an exception for me, their veterinarian, and my assistants. I'm not sure on what basis they make the exception. I have never seen anything about special treatment for veterinarians in the Talmud!" he laughed. "But, you'll see, we will surely get special treatment even if we are dressed in sweaty coveralls and smell like farm animals!"

We climbed into the car and set off.

"Now, you understand," continued Dr. Sirron, "each farmer is like a shareholder in the Hachaklait. The number of shares each farmer has and the amount of his premium depends on the number of cows he has. His premium covers free treatment for each of the cows, veterinary consultations, and payment of eighty percent of the market value of the animal if it dies from illness or accident. But," he shook his bald head, "regardless of how many shares or cows these farmers have, they are all typical Israelis and think that they are the boss, and that we have to dance to their music!

"Our first client in the village is typical — Saadia Cohen, a Yemenite. He owns about five cows and a few calves. But you'd think he paid the biggest premium of anybody in the zone. He complains all the time! Drives me crazy, " sighed Sirron. "He's an interesting guy, though. Skinny like a rail and his *peyot* [sidelocks] are so long they reach down to his neck! He's got two wives, too!" laughed Dr. Sirron. "Imagine that! I have enough trouble with one. Think about two!"

I kept quiet, thinking about this morning's episode with Lina.

"Saadia came with the influx of Yemenites on the 'magic carpet' flight in the early fifties when the majority of Yemenite Jews left Yemen for Israel. Imagine, transported from the dark ages to modern times. He is still close to the dark ages when it comes to cows! He thinks most of what we vets do is magic.

"Today he will be quite put out with me because I didn't come to see his prize cow yesterday. According to Cohen, she's got a big hunk of tissue hanging from her birth canal."

"You mean she's been trying to give birth since yesterday and you didn't go? I'd be put out too! If I had been on call, I would have come immediately."

"Really, Doctor? You'd have been wasting your time!" He laughed. "She already had the calf. This is just the afterbirth which didn't dislodge! You'll have to stop jumping to conclusions if you want to become a good diagnostician!"

I was red faced for having spoken so rashly and for having tried to show off how dedicated I would be as a company doctor. I felt I had flunked my first test with Dr. Sirron.

We drove up to Cohen's small, immaculately kept farm. Saadia and his two wives were waiting for us in the yard between the house and the barn. As predicted, Saadia was furious that Sirron had not come earlier.

"Carmella is my prize cow! If anything happens to her, it's on your head! I have half a mind to write the company about your lack of service!"

"All your cows are prize cows, Saadia," responded Dr. Sirron diplomatically. "And you know perfectly well that this stinking afterbirth could wait until today. You can't rush treatment of a retained placenta. It's like singing *"Eliyahu Hanawi"* [a song customarily sung at the end of the Sabbath] at Friday night services," he said laughing heartily and hugging Saadia with a big bear hug.

"Will you listen to this *chacham gadol* [wise guy]," said Saadia to his wives, wiggling out from Sirron's hug and shrugging his shoulders. They nodded in sympathy and in unison.

"This is my new assistant, Dr. Sorokin," said Dr. Sirron introducing me to Saadia, Zipora, and Miriam. "He comes to us via Italy!" he exclaimed, as though it were some exotic place. I don't think Zipora and Miriam had any idea where Italy was, but they looked appropriately impressed. Saadia looked doubtful. Maybe he had heard stories about the level of practical training of most Italian veterinary students.

"We'll put him to work on your cow if you'll get us a big basin of warm soapy water to clean up in," said Dr. Sirron turning to Miriam, the younger and prettier of the two wives. We all watched as she hurried across the yard to fetch the water — Saadia with pride, and Sirron and I with curiosity. She was dressed in western style clothes, including high heels on which she was barely able to walk. Although modern looking, her clothes were not really coordinated or well fitting, and the colors were garish! In contrast, Zipora, who remained at Saadia's side, looked exactly like a traditional Yemenite woman. She was dressed in a beautifully hand-stitched black robe over harem pants. She and Miriam were quite a contrast of old and new world styles!

Miriam returned and I washed with the soap and water she provided. We all moved to the barn where Carmella, the 'prize' cow was waiting. I struggled into one of the long gloves which covered my entire right arm up to the shoulder. Under Dr. Sirron's supervision, I disgorged the placenta, by now quite soiled on the outside and attracting hundreds of flies. I placed a bolus of antibiotics in the cow's uterus to combat infection and gave her a shot of hormones to help clean up the uterus and eliminate any remnants of the afterbirth. I managed the whole process without a hitch (or a kick from Carmella) and was quite proud of myself. Saadia and his wives watched the entire process intently without ever guessing it was my first time! I hoped Dr. Sirron wouldn't tell them.

"Looks like you have got a real smart assistant this time, Doc," nodded Saadia, "even if he is from Italy. *Ze rofe gaon* [a real genius]," he continued theatrically clapping Sirron on the back. Dr. Sirron smiled in amusement.

"I have heard that most things that come from Italy are of great value, Saadia, maybe even this young doctor is," he said pointing at me. He winked at me, and I knew he wasn't going to spill the beans about this being my first attempt to dislodge an afterbirth.

I smiled in relief. "Well, the only thing that really matters is that Carmella will now feel good and give lots of milk."

"Amen," said Saadia.

"Come, have a coffee now." Miriam entered with the customary Yemenite-style coffee, spiced with *hel* (cardamom). We drank together, Sirron and I making burping sounds to show our appreciation in the Yemenite tradition. Miriam then produced a small plate of *salata matbucha,* a cooked salad which looked just like the dish my mother-in-law used to make. "For you, especially, Doctor," she said shyly.

I couldn't refuse, of course, and quickly swallowed several mouthfuls. I discovered too late that it was spicy and exceedingly hot! With my mouth and stomach burning, I raced for the water faucet near the barn door. Dr. Sirron, Saadia and his two wives enjoyed a good laugh at my expense. I was certain Sirron must have known what I was in for when Miriam offered me the dish. I was really annoyed he hadn't warned me. Well, he probably thought this was part of my training too. Lesson one: Don't be hasty in diagnosis. Lesson two: Eat with caution what your clients offer you! It was only nine o'clock in the morning. I wondered what the rest of the lessons for the day would be!

Sirron spent the next few minutes talking to Saadia about the care of Carmella over the next few days, patiently explaining to him what to expect, what to watch for, and what might warrant another veterinary visit.

"Now don't call us just to show off your beautiful wives!" he chided. "You should be able to take care of this cow from now on if you have paid attention to what I have said!" He patted the cow on the rump and we moved slowly toward the car. It was another fifteen minutes of conversation before we finally left Saadia and his two wives.

"You see," said Sirron in a fatherly tone, "in this job you deal all day with people who have immigrated here, most of whom know nothing about animal husbandry. You must be their teacher as well as their veterinarian, and most of all their friend."

I nodded, but was really thinking about Saadia's two wives and the relationship they had with him. What a difference from Dr. Sirron and Lina!

Our next case was only a short distance away on the small farm of Mr. Imree, a Hungarian immigrant with a bunch of kids (and only one wife!). In contrast to Saadia's place, Imree's was a mess. Both the barn and the house could have used a coat of paint. The yard was unkempt and full of dirty children running around chasing each other. There was a mixture of toys and farm implements strewn about. Even from the car I could tell that the barn obviously had not been swept or really cleaned in weeks. The doors were open and very strong animal odors filled the air. Large piles of straw and muck edged in on either side of the barn doors. Flies swarmed everywhere.

"*Oyoyoi, oyoyoi,*" exclaimed Imree, shaking his dark head and coming to meet us as we stepped out of the car. "*Harbei zaroth* [lots of trouble]," he said in heavily accented Hebrew. He was a tiny, wiry man, with dark skin, eyes and hair. He was dressed neatly, in contrast to the chaos which surrounded him. He looked exhausted. With him was a tall skinny man who introduced himself to me as Lazi, the government-appointed instructor for all the recently arrived Hungarians in the region.

"So what's the trouble?" asked Sirron of Lazi. "Ask him to explain everything in detail."

Turning to me Sirron said, "He's been here for three years and he still doesn't speak enough Hebrew for me to figure out what he's saying!" Lazi conversed in Hungarian with Imree for a few minutes.

"Well, it's simple, but sad," said Lazi. "Five of his ten calves have died this week," said Lazi. "All from diarrhea."

Dr. Sirron looked at me. "Any preliminary thoughts, Doctor?"

"Well, from the looks of this place, I'd say it is probably mostly the result of poor hygiene!"

"Let's have a look around, Lazi," said Dr. Sirron. "I think my assistant has hit it on the head."

We toured the barn, which was indeed filthy. "You tell Imree that even with the most modern antibiotic we can't do a thing to help him if he doesn't clean up this mess!" Turning to Imree directly, Sirron continued, wagging his finger in Imree's face, "This place has got to be cleaner than your house if you want your cows to survive! Such a disgrace. You should be ashamed of yourself with such a barn!" Lazi translated mimicking Sirron's gestures and stern tone of voice.

"Tell him the company will pay for the five dead calves this time, but if he doesn't clean this place up we will cancel his insurance for sure!"

Imree looked properly abashed as he showed us to the pen where the remaining calves were located. "You Hungarians are supposed to be so smart!" Dr. Sirron continued sternly with his lecture to Imree, as we washed up and began to treat the remaining calves. "Any idiot would know better than to try and raise animals in a place as filthy as this! It's a breeding ground for sickness. I'm surprised your own kids aren't sick, too. You'll have to wash this floor down really well and bring in all new straw. And clean out every stall and pen every day!" He was speaking so fast and so furiously that Lazi had a hard time keeping up with him.

"What do you think, Dr. Sorokin" Sirron asked me. "Will these remaining calves make it?"

"Yes," I responded, "I think we're in time with the treatment, if Imree here will follow your advice and clean the place up really well!" I shook my head at the mess, wondering if he would do it.

"Hear that, Imree," said Sirron as if Imree could understand Hebrew. "If these calves die, it's on your head!"

We concluded the visit with detailed instructions for Lazi so he would be able to make sure Imree understood how to give the sick calves the proper care and attention in the next critical hours. Needless to say, we turned down the ritual offer of coffee for obvious reasons. The house didn't look much better than the barn and neither of us wanted to take chances!

"You know, Sorokin," said Dr. Sirron as we drove to the next client. "It's absolutely amazing about these Hungarian Jews. They simply can't seem to learn Hebrew. You know the government tried an experiment here not so many years ago. They settled one Yemenite farmer who spoke Hebrew and Arabic only next to a Hungarian farmer, then another Yemenite, then another Hungarian, and so on. Within three years, all the Yemenites spoke Hungarian and the Hungarians still only spoke Hungarian!"

The next case required minor surgery. The farm was owned by Mania, a very old lady, who essentially ran the place herself. Her husband was still alive, but very ill. She greeted us from the door of her dilapidated old house. She was dressed in faded but clean work clothes, with her snow-white hair almost completely covered with a handkerchief.

"Oh, I'm so glad you are here, Doctor. Betsy has cut her tit on a rusty wire. It's bleeding and I can't milk her. That quarter of her udder is full and she's in misery!"

"Well, we will see what we can do for her, Mania," said Dr. Sirron soothingly.

"This is my assistant, Doctor Sorokin," he said introducing me. "Good thing I have him along today. I have a feeling he will be needed for this job! As I recall Betsy is not the most patient of your cows." He turned and smiled at me as Mania started to protest his comment about Betsy. "Mania thinks all of her cows are part of her family. If you say anything bad about them she gets upset!"

"By the way, speaking of family," he said, turning back to Mania. "How's that husband of yours doing? Still in the hospital?"

"Yes, I don't think he'll be coming home, Doc," she said with tears brimming. She shook her frail, snow-white head and got control of herself. "I don't really know what to do. You know the fact that Betsy got cut is really my fault. I haven't the strength anymore to clean the barn right and make sure no loose baling wire falls in the pens or on the floor."

We walked over to the barn. While it was not neat, it was far cleaner than Imree's place. I was amazed that Mania was able to keep it in such relatively good condition given her age and strength.

Dr. Sirron edged his big body around to Betsy's side in the narrow stall. He patted her side and sat down on the small milking stool to prep her tit with water, phisohex, iodine solution and alcohol. Betsy moved uneasily in the stall, looking over her shoulder at Dr. Sirron and me. "Sorokin, you hold her tail straight in the air. As far up as you can get it. It will hurt her a little, but it will distract her from the pain of the surgery."

"Don't worry," I said reassuringly to Mania, who looked doubtful. "I'll be careful. I know this cow means a lot to you!" Mania smiled weakly.

Contrary to expectations, or perhaps because of my distracting touch, Betsy turned out to be a pretty good patient. She mooed deeply when injected with the local anesthetic, but otherwise didn't seem to notice much. Dr. Sirron freshened and scraped the injured tissue and stitched up the wound with a special figure eight stitch I had never seen before.

"This type of stitch holds well and also allows some give when the area swells up a little right after the surgery," explained Dr. Sirron. "It won't tear as easily as other types of stitches. Okay," he said patting Betsy on the side as he slid by her to get out of the stall. "We're done."

"Oh, thank you so much, doctors," exclaimed Mania. "I was beside myself. You know I can't stand to see animals in pain!" She shook both our hands vigorously.

As usual, the visit ended with the dispensing of medicine and advice and coffee. "Remember, Mania, an ounce of prevention is better than a pound of cure," lectured Dr. Sirron. "Hire yourself some help to clean up the barn so your cows won't have any more of these accidents which can seriously affect their health!"

Mania nodded. "I guess you are right, Doc. But, I hate to spend the money, especially when I don't have it, and most of the help is worthless anyway these days."

"Still better than you trying to do everything yourself, *motec* [sweetheart]," admonished Sirron as he gave her a farewell hug. "You deserve a little help at your age!"

We drove on to the next client, a kibbutz in the next village which was a number of miles away. "You'll see a big difference now in organization and mechanization, Sorokin," remarked Dr. Sirron as we drove through the countryside on the rough, dry road. "These collectives are becoming quite modern. Of course, there's still the problem that many of the people have absolutely no background in farming or animal husbandry. You know, in this job you have to be one part teacher, one part psychiatrist, and one part veterinarian. And sometimes even a policeman. I've run across some really bad cases of animal neglect on some of the smaller farms!"

"Well, yes, I suppose that's bound to happen," I replied, "when you have all these people with good intentions and not much else trying to become farmers overnight!"

"Right you are, Doctor. Well, watching you this morning, I noticed you seem to have the right touch with the human part of our practice. I think you'll be fine once we get a few hundred hours of real field practice behind you. Now this next place will be a good test of your veterinary skill. We will be doing pregnancy testing on about thirty cows. Let's see how fast you get the hang of it."

Max, the barn man, met us as we arrived. "You'll stay for lunch after you're through, won't you, Doc?" asked Max barely before we got out of the car. "What will you have, steak or chicken? I have to let the kitchen know now!"

"Let's have steak, Max. I have a new assistant with me today. He needs strength! Tell them to make some spaghetti, too. He's been in Italy for six years and misses the pasta!" Dr. Sirron laughed, "I don't want you to feel like a stranger in a strange barn, my *dottore italiano.*" It was already past one o'clock and I was starved. I was ready to settle for anything, pasta or not.

Max was a short man with a large belly, a *Yeke*, or German immigrant, who lived up to the stereotype. He was hardworking, but stubborn: he ran the barn like his own small kingdom, or perhaps like an army training camp. His boots were covered with dry cow manure and he wore a very earnest expression.

"Max has been with this kibbutz from the start," explained Dr. Sirron after he introduced me. "He can take real pride in what has been created here. Remember what it was like at the beginning, Max?"

"How can I forget it! This place was a bunch of rocks, weeds, brush and mosquitos. Most of the original members of the kibbutz died from malaria. About half of those who survived left to work in the city. Some even returned to Europe. They couldn't take the hard life here. Luckily, Wilhelmina, a non-Jewish German colony, was located just next to us. They were real farmers. Although I was raised in a city and knew nothing about farming, I at least could speak German and learn from those guys. They were great teachers. Now we have surpassed them! Imagine. Well enough storytelling. I don't want to keep you from your work!" Max went off to give the kitchen the lunch menu for the visiting veterinarians and we began to work.

Dr. Sirron and I each donned a set of coveralls and one shoulder-length glove. "I will test this one first," he said, "while you hold her tail and listen to me explain what to do. Then you will retest her and we shall compare what we think."

With that, he unceremoniously put his gloved hand into the cow's rectum. "First we scoop out the feces until the rectum is empty. A hand-ful at a time. After that we can feel for the uterus through the rectum wall. You need to feel for a squishy fluid contents in the uterus. That's a good sign that the cow is pregnant. Now you have to do this all very care-fully. The embryo is very fragile. If you squeeze too hard you will cause an abortion and Max, our good *Yeke* friend here, will get very upset. Next you search for both ovaries. They are located just behind the kidneys. If the cow is really pregnant the ovaries will feel like a giant lima bean with a wart on top.

"Let me tell you my little secret. I always do this testing with my eyes closed. It helps me to concentrate. Try it yourself. I'll bet it works for you, too.

"Okay," said Dr. Sirron removing his arm from the cow. "Try your luck with this cow now that I have completed my examination. Let's see if we agree on whether or not she's pregnant."

I thrust my arm into the cow and felt for the uterus and ovaries as he had instructed me, keeping my eyes closed and feeling very carefully with my hands. "She's pregnant!" I exclaimed excitedly. "I'm sure of it!"

"Congratulations, Doctor! You're absolutely correct. Now let's get going with the rest of the group."

We spent the next two and one half hours testing each cow. First Dr. Sirron, then I. To my delight, I was right on all but one! That one had fluid in the uterus, but it was the result of an infection, not pregnancy, and I mistook a small bump on one of the ovaries for the corpus luteum.

"So, twenty-nine out of thirty correct. Not bad for your first time out," said Dr. Sirron. "You got the knack of it quite nicely."

It was two-thirty by the time we finished. My arm ached, but I felt good about how quickly I had learned the procedure. We walked over to the kibbutz dining hall for lunch.

Now within a kibbutz, everyone, at least in theory, is equal. Everyone works and receives what he needs to live. No money changes hands. The food is simple and plain. I was somewhat surprised, therefore, to see the size of the steaks that awaited us when we arrived at the dining hall.

Max must have noted my amazement. "Oh, we don't eat like this ourselves, Doctor. This is special for you and Dr. Sirron. We know we get better service if we feed you well!"

Dr. Sirron laughed. "These guys keep their communist-socialist ideals within the kibbutz family! They need me and they know I give them excellent service. They also know a good steak with all the trimmings goes a long way with me!

"A nice arrangement," I smiled, my belly nicely full.

In the car a few minutes later, Dr. Sirron continued. "You know, a member of this kibbutz wouldn't see that kind of steak until his or her seventy-fifth birthday, and most of them don't live that long! But, for the veterinarians that keep their cows healthy, it's pretty much regular fare on every visit! They want us in super shape!"

It was almost four by the time we left the kibbutz and the sun was starting to make its descent behind the mountains into the sea. During the dusty, twenty minute drive Dr. Sirron explained, "Our last stop will be at a small farm owned by an old farmer named Ovadia. I was there last Friday. Ovadia has only one cow. Looks like a skeleton now. I checked her over but wasn't sure of the diagnosis. I told him I would be back today for a recheck. We will let you handle that and then we'll discuss the diagnosis together."

I suspected Dr. Sirron was surer of the diagnosis than he let on. Treating me as if I were his "consultant" was just another way of checking on my diagnostic skill.

Ovadia was waiting for us in his barn, alone with his one cow. His skin was so dark, leathery and wrinkled that he looked like a little raisin. He was stoop-shouldered and skinny and he looked sad. "Your medicine didn't help, doctor. She still won't eat. Look at her, just skin and bones. That medicine was for the birds!"

Dr. Sirron whispered to me, "It was just a placebo. To give Ovadia something to do."

"Psychiatry, again, eh," I whispered back.

"Nachon [right]!," he responded with a smile.

"Well, I brought my assistant this time, Ovadia," said Dr. Sirron. "Between the two of us, we will find out what the problem is. Why don't you go over all the symptoms again for Dr. Sorokin's benefit?"

Ovadia dutifully repeated the list of symptoms, interjecting every now and then how much he loved the cow, how long he had owned her, how much milk she had produced over the years. . . .

I pulled on yet another arms-length glove over my very tired arm and began my examination under Dr. Sirron's watchful eye. After a moment I could start to feel small little nodules high up in the intestinal tract. Little bigger than pea size, most of them. I looked at Dr. Sirron.

"Small tumors, throughout the tract. Progressing downward."

"And the size?"

"Like a small pea or maybe a lima bean, most of them; but there are a few larger ones."

"Hmm. Let me check now," said Dr. Sirron. He pulled on a glove and felt for the same nodules.

"They have grown since Friday. Substantially. It's pretty clear now, eh?" he said looking at me.

"Yes," I responded, "cancer."

"A terrible thing, cancer. Our biggest medical challenge, and we have yet to make any real progress." He shook his head and turned to Ovadia who was standing a short distance away.

"I'm sorry, my friend," he said gently putting his hand on Ovadia's shoulder. "Your cow has cancer which is progressing rapidly. There is nothing we can do. She cannot be saved. We cannot even salvage the meat. Tomorrow the company will send someone to pick her up. You'll receive your compensation check in about a week."

"Nothing you can do?" repeated Ovadia shaking his head and moving over to put his arms around the poor cow's neck. Tears started streaming down his face. "She's been such a good cow. Such a good cow."

We left Ovadia in the barn. "Life and death in the same day, Sorokin," said Sirron in a matter-of-fact tone. "You'll have to get used to it."

The sun was getting low in the purple sky as we left Ovadia's farm and by the time we arrived home the moon and stars were already on duty in the heavens.

"Be sure you really clean up before you come in," shouted Lina from the kitchen window, "I can't stand a double dose of cow manure! And, you, *dottore italiano,* be sure and wash your hair, too. The smell gets in there as well. Naftali, of course, doesn't have that problem since he's so bald," she laughed.

Dinner was delicious and I tried to shower Lina with as many compliments as possible without overdoing it. But it was clear that my refusal this morning was still a sore spot with her. I fervently hoped things would calm down and that she wouldn't press the matter further during my stay! I had really grown fond of Dr. Sirron during our first full day together. He had a wonderful way with animals and their owners. He was totally dedicated to his profession! I simply couldn't stand to let Lina get in the way of my working with him.

The weeks flew by. Dr. Sirron and I left every day at daybreak and returned after dark. I was thrilled with the variety of work I was doing under his guidance. His confidence in me grew as we worked together, treating or testing cows, cows and more cows in addition to a few horses and sheep. By the end of the month he was regularly sending me out on my own to handle cases, while he went to Haifa to meetings at the Hachaklait headquarters.

Finally, the last week of my internship arrived. We were back at the kibbutz where Max, the *Yeke,* was in charge of the barn. "Can't understand it, Doc. The cows are generally off their feed and milk production is down. And now this one picks up a limp from out of nowhere."

I was puzzled as I examined the cow's foot, which was obviously very tender, but without any sign of trauma or a cut. I saw Dr. Sirron frowning as Max recounted the symptoms in greater detail. Suddenly one of the kibbutz members ran into the barn. "Dr. Sirron, there is an urgent phone call for you from Hachaklait headquarters. You can take it up in the main office."

Sirron strode quickly to the kibbutz administrative office and returned a few minutes later looking grim. "We've got a war on our hands, my friends!"

"What!" we all shouted. "Where? Who attacked?"

"No, no, not that kind of war. A veterinary war. Hoof-and-mouth disease. There's been a bad outbreak and all the veterinarians in the country have been mobilized to help treat it and stop the spread of the disease. I'm pretty sure that's what's wrong with these cows, Max."

We began to examine more of the cows in the barn. Sure enough, there were small sores and blisters developing in the mouths of several of the cows.

"What do we do, Doc?" asked Max. "We can't afford to lose these cows, and a low milk production is just about as bad!"

"Well, this is a tough disease to control once it gets started, Max," I responded. "It's a virus. There is no real cure for it."

"No cure!" exclaimed Max. "My God!"

"But," interjected Dr. Sirron, "if we're lucky, we'll be able to save the herd. Starting immediately you must thoroughly clean the stalls and the rest of the barn. Put big pans of lysol near the doors. Don't let anyone in or out without first stepping in the lysol. Feed the cows a real mushy meal for the next couple of weeks. Then, as soon as they are able to tolerate it, gradually work back up to their regular feed. Dr. Sorokin will give you some antibiotics to help fight off secondary infections. In a week or so we should know whether the herd will be saved. The key factor is to keep them eating something. Your milk production is going to be low for sometime, I'm afraid.

"The kibbutz is now under quarantine, Max," said Dr. Sirron sternly. "No new cows should be brought in and none of those that are here can be sold or moved off the property until the disease is contained. You will have to organize a lysol "bath" for your cars and trucks too. No one should enter or leave the property in a vehicle that has not been driven through that "bath" of lysol and water. We don't want the disease to spread from one place to another through the tires of vehicles. And no visitors to the kibbutz, period!"

We provided Max with the medicine he would need for the next week, knowing that we would not have time to return to check on the cows for at least that time. We then hopped in the car and, after about an hour's drive, we reported ourselves at the Beth Dagon Government Research Center, the designated command center for the massive undertaking to fight the onset of hoof-and-mouth disease. The Research Center was surrounded by sweet smelling orange groves. The aroma was overwhelming. The parking lot was full of cars with the familiar green emblem of the Israeli veterinary association.

"It looks as though every veterinarian in the country is here," I exclaimed.

"Yes, or they will be before long," replied Dr. Sirron.

The Research Center building itself was gleaming white, reflecting the sun so as to almost blind you as you approached the massive doors. I had not noticed Dr. Shoshan, my old boss from the Department of Agriculture, until I almost ran into him at the entrance.

"So, Yehudale," he exclaimed shaking my hand. "You see you can't escape vaccinations even at the Hachaklait! Didn't I tell you it is always easier to prevent disease in a thousand cows than to treat one?"

"That you did," I answered with a smile. "However, I still prefer the treatment end to the endless vaccination routine. But, of course, in this case, I am more than willing to spend whatever time is necessary helping out with both vaccinations and treatment."

We went inside to the central hall where chairs had been set up as in a theater for all the veterinarians to attend meetings and to receive instructions as to what needed to be done. Dr. Gur and Dr. Freund gave us an inspirational pep talk on the importance of our mission to prevent the spread of the disease. Two automatic syringes and lots of vaccines were then issued to each of us; we were also given a daily assignment with instructions to complete it "no matter what!" We were each to return to the Research Center within the next few days for additional assignments. The entire country was to be covered!

Within the hour an armada of vehicles left the parking lot, a veterinarian and a helper in each car, armed with maps, syringes, vaccine and a list of locations to be visited.

My first stop was at kibbutz Givat Brenner. The barn supervisor had the whole herd tied up and waiting. The farmers helped hold each cow for inspection and then for the injection with the automatic syringe which was attached by a long tube to a one-liter bottle of vaccine. Within a couple of hours the herd was vaccinated. My helper and I jumped back in the car and headed for the next kibbutz. On the way we ate sandwiches that had been prepared for us at the Research Center. We were so hungry!

We finished three more kibbutzim in the afternoon, vaccinating about six hundred cows. The last stop took longer than the first two because the farmers had not been warned beforehand about the need to round up the cows for the vaccination. So we had to wait while some of them were brought in from an outlying area.

By the end of the day, close to nine o'clock in the evening, we were exhausted, but satisfied that the needed work had been promptly completed. Israel couldn't afford to lose the bulk of its dairy cattle, and in such a small country the disease could spread rapidly. Time was critical, so no one complained about the eighteen-hour workdays; by the end of the third day the entire cow population in Israel had been vaccinated.

At the conclusion of the vaccination blitz, Dr. Schturman called me at Dr. Sirron's home. "Go on home to your wife, Dr. Sorokin. Your internship has been completed. Dr. Sirron gives you high marks and we think you're ready to work as a substitute veterinarian in the southern region near your home in Ashkelon. Enjoy a few days off. Early next week your fully equipped company car will be delivered and you'll be ready to go! *Mazal Tov,* good luck!"

I hung up the phone and rushed to my room to pack. I was so excited I even hugged Lina and gave her a big kiss on the forehead. "You were a great hostess," I cried to the surprised Lina as I rushed down to the garage to say my farewells to Dr. Sirron who was still puttering in his workshop.

"Well, I've got my first assignment," I reported excitedly to Dr. Sirron. "Starting next week, I'm the official substitute vet for the southern region. I can't thank you enough for all you have taught me during the last month. It was an honor to have worked with you!"

"Well, I'll say this," said Dr. Sirron with a smile. "You're the best spaghetti vet I ever had for an intern! I know you'll do well. Enjoy your few days off. Once you start practice in earnest, those free days are few and far between."

We shook hands and I drove off in my old Opel, dreaming of the new car that would soon be mine, and of the position it would represent. Full-time field veterinarian at last!

XVIII

The Horse Who Came to Seder

✳

I t was a wonderful time to be in Israel. National pride in our victory in the '56 war was still strong, despite international political pressure that threatened to reduce Israel's hard-fought gains. A new generation of sabras, born to survivors of the Holocaust, began to fill the streets and schools — chattering noisily in Hebrew, a language their immigrant parents had not yet mastered (and which many of them never would).

Government efforts to build a nation out of the diverse social and ethnic population continued, occasionally with amusing results, as when the Yemenites learned Hungarian instead of the Hungarians learning Hebrew! Despite ethnic jokes and rivalries, failed experiments, misunderstandings and miscalculations, there was a sense of commitment to Israel, as if we all knew that, in time and with hard work, the dream would become reality.

Time and hard work! My own job as a replacement veterinarian took both. I was determined to excel so that my own personal dream would become a reality: a veterinary region of my very own. We continued to live in Ashkelon, but I was constantly on the road replacing one or another assigned veterinarian during his vacation or sick leave.

"You are never home!" complained my wife. "I'm starting to think you care more about cows than you do about your family!" Of course, this wasn't true, but in retrospect I understand that it could have seemed so to her. I was pursuing my dream: up at dawn and working well into the evening, driving around the province in my pride and joy: a new green station wagon provided by the Hachaklait. When I left each morning, loaded up with my medicines and veterinary equipment, I felt like Don Quixote riding off on Rosinante to conquer the terrible foe.

"I hope you're not planning to work on *Erev Pesach,* Yehudale," chided my wife a few nights before Passover. "You know we are having forty people for the first night Seder and I could really use your help the entire day!"

"Don't worry," I laughed. "In Israel, the animals never get sick on Seder night. No one will need me. I will be home to help." She looked at me with dubious eyes, knowing full well that I wasn't taking her concerns very seriously.

And sure enough, at four-thirty in the morning on Passover eve our phone rang. It was Abi, the newly trained *madrich* (advisor) to the village of Kfar Achim, a new settlement of mostly Eastern European Jews. "We've got a real emergency, Doc. One of my newest farmers, recently arrived from the meadows of downtown Budapest, gave his cow some wet alfalfa last night. She's blown up like a balloon."

"Some advisor you are, Abi. You're supposed to teach these people how to take care of their animals, not how to kill them off!"

"Come on, Doc. They just arrived and I can't watch over them every second. Better hurry, though. It looks pretty serious to me."

"Don't worry," I said to my wife as I hurriedly started off, "I'll be back in plenty of time to help you for tonight."

The sun was just coming up and the sea was absolutely calm as I left Ashkelon. The sweet scent of orange blossoms filled the air as I passed the orange groves on the edge of town. Soon the scenery changed to green fields dotted with small cow barns and black and white Swiss Holsteins. The odor of fresh cow manure replaced the smell of orange blossoms. Strangely, I almost preferred it!

Everything was peaceful. The cows were quietly munching at the long wooden troughs filled with hay. Little black birds perched on their backs, picking off the ticks for breakfast.

Abi was waiting for me as I turned off the road into the small village. He was quite a figure: a dark Yemenite with long, meticulously groomed sidelocks, and wearing his *Kova Tembel*, the traditional Israeli hat, even at this early hour of the morning in this little country village (religious Jews wear hats at all times).

"These big-city Hungarians are good at making goulash, Doctor," he said, as he lead me to Lazlo's barn. "but they have no idea about how to take care of cows! I guess they think cows can eat anything."

From inside the barn we could hear loud shouting in Hungarian. "Lazlo and his wife," explained Abi, "each blaming the other for this disaster."

They grew silent as we entered, concern over the cow taking precedence over the argument now that the doctor had arrived. Deggi, Lazlo's wife, was dispatched to the kitchen to bring me the *sappoon* and *turrilkusse* (soap, water and towels in Hungarian) I needed to prepare for the job of trying to save their cow. I washed quickly while Abi showed Lazlo how to put the cow's head into a head restraint and how to use the special nose gripper to help keep the cow under control.

"We have to act fast," I said to Abi. " This cow is on its last legs." Despite the head restraint and Lazlo's efforts with the nose gripper, the cow was still moving about some. "Deggi, please lift the cow's tail hard," I ordered, gesturing to make myself understood as I wasn't too sure about her Hebrew. "This will help restrain her, too. But stand back when you do it," I added quickly, turning my attention to the cow which was now standing still. Unfortunately, Deggi didn't understand this last admonition and planted herself right up against the cow's rear end. Abi was just starting to warn her when she jumped back with a scream, her neck, shoulder and arm covered with a messy green substance which had sprayed forth from the cow's rectum. We all tried not to laugh, but she certainly was a sight! Deggi, however, was so concerned about the cow she ignored us and, barely taking the time to clean up, immediately resumed her assigned task, although this time from a respectful distance and slightly to one side.

While Lazlo held the cow's head and Deggi its tail, Abi and I opened its mouth and forced a long plastic tube into its stomach. "We'll see if this works," I said. "If not I'll have to use the trocar (a sort of hollow dagger in a sheath) and stab a hole in her side for the gas to escape." A foul odor permeated the air as small amounts of gas started to pass through the stomach tube.

I shook my head after a few minutes.

"It's not enough. The tube isn't reaching enough of the gas to give her relief." Lazlo shouted in dismay as I picked up my trocar and headed toward the cow's side.

"He thinks you're going to kill her to put her out of her misery," explained Abi.

"Tell him not to worry," I laughed. "This stabbing is meant to save her life. And if I don't do this, she'll die on her own and in very short order!"

I reached down and swiftly drove the trocar into the triangle of the cow's flank, deep into her belly. I pulled it out, leaving the sheath to serve as a passage for the gas to escape. Instantly, enormous amounts of foul-smelling gas and bubbly fluid gushed out, deflating her like a balloon that had been popped. The crisis was over. I gave her shots of antibiotics and atropin to wind up my victory over the bloat.

"*Ata rope ala kefak*," commented Abi in an amusing mixture of Hebrew and Arabic meaning, more or less, "You're a terrific vet, by the grace of God."

Deggi disappeared into the house and returned with a tray of Hungarian breakfast goodies, including bacon, freshly baked bread, and steaming syrupy coffee. Abi accepted the coffee, but moved away from us quickly, shaking his head at "these Woos Wouses" (a nickname for European Jews) who offended God's law by eating pig in the Holy Land, especially on the eve of Passover.

I loved the bacon and bread, but was careful to turn away from Abi while eating it, and tried to smooth over the offence by praising his good work with the settlers.

Abi was perfectly willing to have his attention diverted to the subject of his genius in working with new immigrants. After basking in my compliments, he asked, "Say, while you're here, Doc, how about visiting some of the other farmers? They really need all the education and advice we can give them. And they'll pay more attention when the advice comes from a real doctor. Let's not let the opportunity go to waste."

I laughed, easily diverted from my promise to return home to help my wife. "I can see why the government put you in this job, Abi. You are really dedicated! Of course, I'll stay if you think I can be of help to you."

We spent the rest of the morning visiting with most of the village farmers, dispensing a little medicine and lots of advice and trading stories about former homelands and the sometimes painful, sometimes funny, process of adapting to new life in Israel.

My wife was hard at work on the Seder meal when I arrived home in the early afternoon. "How convenient of that cow to get sick just when I need you at home to help!" she commented as I entered. "I hope you are ready to work here now."

"Sure, sure," I replied. "Just give me thirty minutes to take a nap. I've been up since four-thirty in the morning you know."

My wife rolled her eyes and shook her head. "You'll never change. I know it will be a cold day in Hell before I get any help out of you around the house!" But her annoyance at my late arrival and desire for a nap was somewhat eased by the dozen eggs I brought with me, a gift from one of the farmers I had spent some time with in the morning. Eggs were still fairly hard to get and we were going to need a lot of them in order to make eighty matzah balls that night.

The first night Seder was always an eagerly awaited event in our small household. We weren't religious, but we both had a strong sense of Jewish tradition instilled in us by our parents. And Passover was one of the most cherished traditions, the celebration of the Jews' escape from Egypt and slavery.

Passover was one of the few occasions when my wife's orthodox upbringing would surface. She loved all the traditional ceremonies. Our house, which was always clean, would literally sparkle after the extra cleaning in preparation for Passover. Little Fafa helped with the Bivr Chametz — the ceremony consisting in hiding bread crumbs in prearranged places, so that the crumbs could later be collected and placed in a container for ceremonial burning, symbolizing the removal of non-kosher food from the house. Dishes and pots were cleaned in huge pots over open fires on the streets, making them kosher for Pesach. Even my car had to be washed and cleaned in honor of Passover!

We always invited friends for the first night Seder. This year we had outdone ourselves and invited forty people! The table (actually an assortment of little tables placed next to each other) extended from the kitchen through the living room and down the hall. At the very end of the table was the oversize chair I would use as head of the Seder. It was covered with cushions to recall the tradition that the Seder dinner has to be eaten while reclining.

The table was covered with white bedsheets, since we didn't have enough tableclothes for such a setup! We had borrowed dishes and silverware and nothing matched, but somehow, perhaps because of the decorative flowers my wife had beautifully arranged, everything looked very festive. And the house smelled wonderful, thanks to the aroma of her cooking.

Much to my wife's disgust, I was pretty useless as a helper even after my nap. Not only was I easily distracted, but I was clearly not committed to the task and complained that I was not suited for "women's work." Finally she banished me to the yard to wash the dog. "Good idea," I said. "I'll make him kosher for Passover, too!"

Sometime later, she called from the kitchen window. "Yehudale, I'm going to take my nap now! The matzah balls are ready and they are perfect this year!" she said proudly. "Don't you dare to eat even one while I'm asleep. I've made just enough for tonight!"

Of course we both knew I could never resist sneaking just one! It was a little game we played every year. "No, of course not," I called back. "Go ahead and take your nap. Your matzah balls are safe!" I then made a beeline for the kitchen. And there, waiting for me on the counter, as I knew it would be, was a small bowl of soup with a gigantic fluffy matzah ball floating in the center. I laughed with delight and quickly ate it up. She was right, the matzah balls were perfect this year.

Sundown approached and our guests began to arrive: relatives, neighbors and friends from all walks of life, farmers, tradesmen, even local officials. Samba, our dog, announced the arrival of each new guest with excited barking and tail wagging. Everyone was dressed up, smiling and talkative. Our small living room was quickly filled to the brim and the noise of greetings and conversation was deafening: "How is your youngest?" "We were so pleased to be invited." "Did you hear about Eva?" "The orange crop will be the best ever this year, you can tell by the. . . ." "Tell me, Doctor, what can I do about the fleas that keep bothering the dog?" "Did you hear that Chaim was shot by a sniper on the road?" Gradually the group drifted into two distinct gatherings, the women talking about family matters and the men about local and national politics.

"Haven't you noticed the parallels between the Hebrews' escape from Egypt in biblical times and Israel's victory over the Egyptians during the 1956 war?" asked Yaacov, the local union head loudly, the center of attention as he undoubtedly intended. "It's really uncanny."

"What are you talking about, Yaacov. You are crazy! When did you see the Red Sea divide recently? You've been in the sun too long."

"No, I know what he's talking about," I exclaimed, jumping into the conversation with zest. "Think about it. In ancient times, the Hebrews were enslaved; then, finally, they won their freedom and were allowed to leave Egypt. But shortly after the freedom was granted, they were nearly annihilated by the Egyptians on the shores of the Red Sea. Their hard-fought freedom was almost lost; if it were not for the intervention of God, who opened the Red Sea and then closed it, drowning the enemy.

"The 1956 war brought us our freedom from the terror of the Egyptian army. This time the Egyptians didn't drown in the Red Sea, they "drowned" in the sands of the Sinai at the hands of our army. But, now, just a year later, we are in danger of losing our freedom again. We have been forced to give back territory we won and a new form of guerrilla warfare has been started by the fedayin, a group sponsored by Egyptians and other Arabs. Why, many of our roads are too dangerous to be used at night now."

"You're right, Yehudale," exclaimed Yoram, the town's lawyer. "Why, think of Chaim shot by a sniper on the road to Be'er Sheva only last week. And I hear there are guerilla groups setting ambushes and traps all along the road leading to the Gaza Strip. Even daytime travel is getting dangerous in the South."

"Enough politics!" exclaimed my wife, "It's time to begin the Seder."

Everyone took their places quickly. Since almost every guest had brought a dish to add to the enormous meal my wife had prepared, the table was almost groaning under the weight of food.

"Ladies and gentlemen," I began my opening Seder speech. "It is indeed with great happiness that we sit with you on this first Seder night. Even if we are a little squeezed at the table, it's better than being alone on such a night as this. Now, as prescribed by tradition, everyone fill a glass with wine to celebrate the festival of liberation from Egyptian slavery and . . ." and the phone rang.

"Oh no," cried little Fafa in dismay, "Some animals must be sick and Daddy will have to leave! That's what always happens when the phone rings!"

"Don't be silly, Fafa," I replied. "I told you animals in Israel never get sick on Seder night."

"But, how can that be," she asked in all seriousness. "How do they know when it's Passover?"

By this time the entire table was quiet, waiting for my answer as my wife returned from the phone. "Someone named Maurice. His horse is sick. He says it's an emergency."

"I told you so," exclaimed Fafa in triumph. I smiled wanely and went to the phone.

"*Adon* Doctor," said Maurice with his Moroccan accent. "I am so sorry to bother you. I know you must be sitting at the Seder table like everyone else in the country. But Dr. Zimbach told me I should call you while he is away on vacation. Jose is my only horse. I think he's going crazy from pain and will die if you don't come immediately!"

"Where are you, Maurice?" I asked, knowing his location was not likely to be close. Dr. Zimbach's region was quite a ways to the South, around Be'er Sheva. "Near Sde-Boker," he replied.

"My God, that's at least an hour away," I exclaimed. "And on the Be'er Sheva road! It's full of fedayin at night. We were just talking about it!"

The whole room was listening to my side of the conversation. "Be'er Sheva!" I heard several guests murmur. "He's not going to try to drive that road tonight? No horse is worth that!"

I was thinking similar thoughts. Hoping to avoid the trip, I started to question Maurice about the symptoms of his horse's illness.

"Well, Doc, he's literally writhing in pain. He's breathing heavily. The skin around his mouth is pale and he's foaming. I don't know what to do!"

"Colic," I thought to myself. "Perhaps we can fix him up by phone, if I can convince Maurice that he can do it himself."

"Well, Maurice, you diagnosed it right. The horse is indeed in trouble. Let's see if you can do as well in treating her. This shouldn't wait for me to arrive an hour or more from now, if by the grace of God I should get by the fedayin."

"*Yerachem Hashem*," responded Maurice, "With God's grace."

"Your horse has acute colic. Here's what you do. Take a full bottle of arack [a very strong alchoholic drink kept in stock in most Moroccan homes]. You hold the horse's upper lip, twisting it with a corded stick, and have your wife pour the *arack* into the horse's mouth — the whole bottle. Then make the horse walk constantly whether he wants to or not. Use your whip if necessary. Call me in half an hour and let's see if he's any better."

Maurice wasn't too happy with the delaying tactic, but the guests at the Seder applauded as I sat down. "Do you think it will work?" "Why *arack*?" "Can you be sure over the phone it's colic and not something else?" "Is horse colic like baby colic?" "What will happen now?" "Could she die?" I was bombarded with questions.

"Let's get on with the Seder," I said. "This may not work and I may have to leave after all in half an hour."

We finished the blessing on the wine. I drank the whole cup, which is more than I usually do, better to face the fear that I might have to tackle the Be'er Sheva road. And I prayed fervently, not just in the Passover tradition, but thinking of Maurice's horse, and my reputation if the recommended treatment didn't work!

We went through all the customary songs and my wife sang the *"Ha Lachma"* in honor of her Sephardic tradition. She had coached Fafa to ask "Why is this night different from the rest of the nights?" and the other three traditional questions. "Excellent, Fafa," I exclaimed. You did as good a job as any son could do!" "But I have another question," she interjected as I prepared to continue the ceremony. "What will happen to the horse in Sde-Boker?"

"Yes," someone else added. "It's been almost half an hour. I wonder how Maurice and the horse are coming along."

"Maybe no news is good news," commented another. Just then the phone rang again.

"*Adon* Doctor," began Maurice. "Jose is now bleeding from the mouth. He is still walking, but swaying like a drunk. I really think you should come!"

"Well, of course, he's swaying like a drunk. He's just had a whole bottle of *arack*. You'd be unbalanced too! Now, listen to me. Get a garden hose, douse her with water, and then take a burlap bag and massage the hell out of her. Call me in fifteen minutes."

"We'll just have time to finish before he calls again," I said trying to cut off the comments.

"Wait a minute," cried several of the guests. "We feel like we know this horse now." "Tell us what's going on!" "Do you still think it's colic?" "Is he any better?" "Why the garden hose and massage?"

I could see my wife looking at me at the other end of the table. I could almost hear her thoughts: "You and your animals! This horse is ruining the Seder!"

I gave her a smile and a sort of "what can I do" shrug, and started to respond to everyone's questions. The horse might just as well have been invited to the Seder!

We barely had finished the ceremony and started on the *gefilte* fish when Maurice called again. The room was absolutely silent as I went to the phone.

"She's vomiting, Doctor. . . ." That was all I had to hear. Horses rarely vomit except at the very end of the line. I would have to go now, fedayin or no.

"Just keep doing what I told you, Maurice. *Ani ba miyad* [I'm coming immediately]." A horrified gasp ran through the guests. Everyone looked terrified.

"The road is so dangerous!" my wife cried.

"Here, let me go with you," said Israel, my neighbor and close friend, as I grabbed my Sten gun from the locked cabinet near the door. "No, no. You have a new baby. There is no sense in endangering two of us. This is my job anyway. Excuse me for leaving you like this," I called to my abandoned guests as I jumped into the car.

I roared out of town into the dark night and on to the Be'er Sheva road, hugging my sten with my right hand and steering with my left. I had the accelerator all the way to the floor and the car sped southward with all the power it could muster. It was just me, my Sten and the car against the invisible foe possibly waiting for me somewhere on the road to Be'er Sheva. I knew I would be like a sitting duck. No matter how fast the car went, it wouldn't be fast enough if an ambush had been set. My car lights would be seen from the distance, but I couldn't turn them off and still drive with the speed I needed to reach Maurice and his dying horse. I would just have to take the risk.

I was driving at a hundred and twenty kilometers an hour, approaching the turn where the Gaza Strip area ends, when I saw some Arabs ahead on the road building a stone barricade. Luckily, it wasn't nearly finished. There would be room to get by. Of course, they saw me just as I saw them. I watched them scatter, their white *kafias* trailing as they ran for cover and, I thought, to get their guns. I opened my window and crouched low in the seat. As I passed the unfinished barricade I unloaded the Sten, everything in the cartridge, into the darkness in the direction I had seen them run. I heard screams and answering fire. I knew my car had been hit, but by a miracle it kept going. I made it through! I was sweating and shivering at the same time. I don't remember the rest of the drive to Sde-Boker. It seemed like a long time.

When I pulled into Maurice's yard he exclaimed "You must have flown! It's been barely forty-five minutes since I called!"

"How is Jose?" I asked fearing the worst.

Maurice broke into a smile. *"Toda raba,* Doctor. He is fine now. I tried to call you but you had already left. You are one terrific phone-doctor!"

I grinned weakly and then sat down, exhausted from the stress of the trip and worry over the horse. I spent the rest of that Seder night with Maurice, his horse and another bottle of *arack!*

XIX

On All Fours

✳

y now we were really at home in Ashkelon. We had made lots of friends among the recent immigrants, and had also been adopted by the elite "old timers," of the city, the South African founders. My wife was putting her beautiful voice to good use as a *chaltures,* sort of an itinerant singer, working for the cultural arm of an organization which arranged for entertainment at various kibbutzim throughout Israel. We spent many a Friday afternoon driving to some remote kibbutz where she would be one of the entertainers for the evening, and her reputation as a singer spread.

I, too, was becoming well known, both for my veterinary skill and for my love for arguing politics with just about anyone who would listen. So, despite our youth and relatively recent arrival in Ashkelon, we played an active role in most of the town's social and political events. We even helped create a few!

One evening my wife and I were sitting in our living room after listening to a radio report on the polio epidemic which was spreading throughout Israel afflicting hundreds of children. "You know," I said, "people don't have much money to give to causes these days, but I bet that if we gave a benefit, where everyone could dress up and show off their finery, we would get a good enough turnout to make a significant contribution to the battle against polio. You could sing, I could emcee, like I did for the Air Force, and tell a few stories . . . and I'm sure you could convince your accompanist friend, Hedva, to donate her talents for the evening, too. What do you think?

Well, a few weeks later, it was all arranged. The big *Bet-Am* (People's House) would be our theater and just about the whole town had promised to attend. In little Ashkelon, this would be the event of the year!

Hedva had agreed to accompany my wife and to play an additional solo as well. Because they had worked together so many times entertaining at different kibbutzim, my wife and Hedva easily agreed upon a program of music with which they were familiar and for which they would need very little rehearsing: a few nostalgic songs from the very early years of Jewish settlement in Palestine, some traditional Jewish and European songs, and several popular arias from classic Italian operas.

"Take good care of Fafa while I'm gone," cried my wife as she left for Hedva's house to practice just three days before the concert. "The baby should sleep the whole time I'm gone if you are not too noisy and don't wake her up!"

Fafa wanted to play "horsey," one of our favorite sports, so I was resigned to spending most of the afternoon down on all fours crawling around the living room with her on my back. Of course, despite the admonition, we were noisy! But luckily the baby slept on.

Suddenly the phone rang. It was my wife.

"Yehudale, you won't believe it! Hedva's hand and arm are swollen terribly. She doesn't think she'll be able to play! Call Izzi to stay with the kids and come right over! We have to think of something! The concert is in three days!"

Luckily, Izzi was home and able to come to watch the kids. Very worried, I jumped into the car, my mind racing. What a predicament! Hedva was my wife's favorite accompanist. Neither of the other two accompanists she used most frequently were as good, and I was pretty sure both were out of town. Without Hedva there would be no concert!

When I knocked, Hedva opened the door with her left hand. Her right hand was in a sling and looked red and swollen. She shook her head sadly. "I've been hoping and praying that Dr. Horowitz would find the solution to this mysterious swelling," she said. "It just came on suddenly last week. I didn't call you any earlier because I was certain I would be well enough to play by now. But you can see how swollen my arm is. I'll never be able to do it."

"Yehuda, you can fix her up, can't you? I know you can!" cried my wife in desperation. "You must have something in those medicines you carry around that can be useful." Turning to Hedva, she added, with some exaggeration, "He has helped out many of our friends before." Hedva looked astounded and definitely somewhat dubious.

"But, Dr. Horowitz has tried all week. He even sent me to a specialist in Tel Aviv. Nothing works."

"Yehuda, can do it! I know it," repeated my wife, showing more confidence in my medical skill than I ever thought she had.

"Well, I can try," I said. "After all, you have some similarities to some of my patients," I teased Hedva. "But, you'll have to promise not to say a word to anybody, especially not to Dr. Horowitz! If he found out that I helped you after he was unable to, it would be a scandal! These medical doctors are a jealous lot and they don't take kindly to others messing around in their business. I'm not so sure what the Hachaklait would say, either. But, we have to do something to try and save the benefit for the kids."

"I wouldn't tell a soul" replied Hedva. "I just want to be well enough to play at the concert!"

After a few questions to Hedva about the nature of her pain and the onset of the swelling, I went to the car and pulled out a big jar of horse liniment and some gauze bandages. I rubbed the liniment all over Hedva's arm and hand, bandaged her up and said, "Well, Hedva, this very often works on sore limbs of cows and horses. Let's see if it works on pianists! It can't hurt you anyway, and maybe it will help. Keep it bandaged and call me in twenty-four hours."

Three days later, Hedva and my wife got a standing ovation for their efforts at the benefit. The entire audience, dressed to the nines in long gowns and tuxedos which rarely saw the light of day in little Ashkelon, applauded and stamped their feet, demanding encore after encore. At the reception following the concert, only Dr. Horowitz looked unhappy. I saw him headed my way and guessed that Hedva must have talked!

"You there, Dr. Sorokin," I heard him call as I tried to dissappear into the crowd. "I want to talk to you! Can't you stick to your cows? Hedva now thinks you cured her with that horse liniment and that my efforts failed. She has told everyone! I'm the laughing stock of the whole town! Just look around you, everyone here is talking about it!"

Sure enough, you could hear it throughout the room. . . ."Did you know Yehuda rubbed her arm with horse liniment and immediately the swelling went down?" "I heard old Horowitz was baffled, and here's this upstart vet who cures his patient, quick as a flash. . . ."

"Sorry, Abe," I replied. "I didn't mean any harm, and besides, who knows what really caused that swelling to go down? Anyway, for the sake of this benefit, I would have done the same thing even if it had been your wife whose arm was swollen. . . ."

"You keep away from my wife!" he said heatedly, turning on his heel and giving numbers of people around us the wrong impression of what we had been discussing!

Word of my "medical miracle" inevitably reached the administrative offices of the Hachaklait. As predicted, the senior officers were officially quite unamused, although I'm told in private that even Dr. Schturman thought the incident was quite funny.

I got an official warning, nonetheless. "Stick to your job, Dr.

Sorokin. Leave the two-legged animals to the MDs! We have enough trouble with you trying to out-do all the veterinarians you substitute for. Don't take on the medical profession, too!"

Now, climbing the ladder in the Hachaklait in those days was dependent both on what you knew and whom you knew, together with a bit of luck. Through hard work I was making a name for myself as a good veterinarian among the Hachaklait clientele. In addition, my escapades with the *fedayin* on Seder night and most recently the incident with Dr. Horowitz, helped keep my name in the forefront of the administration's members' mind. I knew that at least I would not be overlooked in the bureaucracy! Good, permanent jobs in the Hachaklait were hard to come by, and I was resigned to being a substitute vet out of Ashkelon for quite some time.

Shortly after the benefit, however, Dr. Schturman called to announce that the vet in Gedera was leaving for eight months as he was on loan to the Israeli government to supervise the importation of cattle from Yugoslavia. "If everything we hear about you is true, and not just your own good PR job," said Schturman, "you should be ready to serve as his full-time replacement." I was ecstatic. This would almost be like having my own post.

"Now, remember, however, my fine Italian doctor," admonished Dr. Schturman, "that we expect you not only to do a good job as a veterinarian, but to keep from criticizing your elders. And no showing off, if you know what's good for you. Be there next week. We will pay the rent on a house for you in Gedera and you can rent out your place in Ashkelon for the eight months and keep the income.

"Yes, sir! You can count on me!" I replied quickly, ignoring what I considered unfair jabs at my behavior.

My wife, however, was definitely not ecstatic. "We just got settled here," she wailed with tears streaming down her face. "I just started to really feel at home and part of the community!"

"Yes," cried little Fafa, taking her cue from her mother. "Why do we have to leave now? I have so many good friends here and everybody loves Mom's singing. Can't we stay, please?" Tears welled up in her eyes, too.

"Hey, we will make new friends! You'll see," I said trying to comfort her. "And Mom can sing in Gedera just as well as in Ashkelon. Don't worry! Everything will be all right."

I could see that I hadn't convinced either of them. Finally, I gave up on consolation, shrugged my shoulders and said, "Well, that's how it is. I worked hard to become a veterinarian and this is my first big break.

We have to take it! I need your support. Let's put the tears behind us and pack. We have only got one week to get things in order."

It didn't help the transition that our house in Gedera was a far cry from the one in Ashkelon. The Gedera home was enormous by Israeli standards and surrounded by towering eucalyptus trees, but it had no view of the sea, and more importantly, we had to share the place with another family. The house wasn't really designed for two-family living and we were constantly running into our fellow tenants. Gradually, though, we adjusted to the lack of privacy and learned to almost enjoy the "communal" living.

Our fellow tenants were the Von Weisel family, known for their far- right political views. The elder Von Weisel was a professor of history of Zionism and the right-hand man of the famous Vladimir Jabotinsky, leader of the extreme right-wing Zionist party of Israel. Von Weisel was really quite a character. He always had his nose in a book. Indeed he was notorious for missing buses because he would become so engrossed in what he was reading. One after another bus would pass him by until someone would notice him still at the station late in the morning and tap him on the shoulder. "Professor Von Weisel, didn't you want to take the early bus to Tel Aviv?"

"Oh my goodness, yes!" he would reply. "I just got so involved in this book. . . ."

I relished the opportunity to discuss politics with him on the nights we were both at home. I was still an advocate of pure socialism, while he was certain that capitalism and free enterprise were essential for the growth of Israel. We would argue and discuss long into the night, a wel- come diversion for me from my long days spent with cows and horses and, especially, farmers who barely knew enough to keep their animals alive and well.

Those discussions really were just a diversion. My passion was not Zionism or socialism or capitalism. It was veterinary medicine and help- ing the unbelievable mixture of immigrants learn to survive and prosper in the vastly different world in which they found themselves, a world in which their old ways would not always work.

A number of my veterinary problems in Gedera were related to those traditional ways which didn't work as well in Israel as they had in the "old country." For example, every week the cows at the ultra-orthodox kibbutz near Gedera would have an attack of mastitis (inflammation of the udder). In this case, the disease was brought on by the practice of having a *shabes goy*, that is, a non-Jew, help with essential tasks on the Sabbath. The ultra-orthodox do not work on the Sabbath, except in emergencies to save a life. But, long ago, a tradition developed among them to hire non-Jews to help out with certain essential tasks which were otherwise forbidden to the Jews. Now milking, although essential for the health of the cow, was not considered within the allowed Sabbath exceptions, so the members of Kibbutz Nezach Yisrael relied on the *shabes goy* tradition. But in Israel the only *goyim* around were Arabs, mostly uneducated and certainly not experienced in modern milking techniques. No experience had prepared them for the importance of thoroughly cleaning both the cow's udder and the cups of the milking machine before hooking up the milking apparatus. Unaccustomed to milking by machinery, they had no concept that the machine could actually milk the cows dry if not removed in time. Try as he would, Joshua, the barn supervisor at the kibbutz, didn't seem able to get these chores through to his Arab shabes goyim, and so I would be summoned every Sunday to deal with the inevitable mastitis.

"*Reb Joshua,*" I would shake my finger at him every week. "This is not doing your cows any good! You've got to train your workers better!" But Joshua would just shrug his shoulders, his long sidelocks dangling from both sides of his head.

"We do the best we can, Doc," he would always answer, slowly stroking his long salt and pepper colored beard. "But, you know it's tough. These *goyim* just don't seem to get the hang of it. There's nothing else I can do. It's hard to be Jewish, you know. But God will have mercy! *Yerachem Hashem.*"

"I can't believe God wants your cows to be sick every week, Joshua! Are you sure there's no way for you to handle the milking on the Sabbath?"

"God forbid," was his inevitable reply.

"And God give me the patience to accept the things I cannot change," were my parting thoughts each week as I walked to my car, knowing that I would be back again next Sunday.

I worked long days in Gedera. Despite the admonition I had received from Dr. Schturman, I was determined not just to excel, but to surpass Dr. Fertig, the veterinarian I was replacing, in providing service to the local clients of the Hachaklait. I was so much younger than he that my credibility was initially somewhat suspect among my clients. Everyone called me "the young doctor," a label which irritated me no end!

One of my first clients in Gedera was Mr. Yakobovitch, a Rumanian Jew who first introduced himself to me shortly after we arrived in town by telephoning me at about two o'clock in the morning. I was soundly asleep, exhausted after a long day which had begun before dawn.

When the phone rang, I confused the shrill sound with that of my alarm clock and tried to ignore it! "Too early to get up!" I murmured. But the sound wouldn't stop! Gradually it dawned on me that it was the telephone and I stumbled out of bed and into the hall to answer it.

"About time someone answered!," exclaimed a voice with a strong Rumanian accent. "Is this the young doctor? I need you right away. I have an emergency!"

"Well, I'm the doctor, though not so young anymore," I replied, automatically giving my standard retort and silently thinking that at the rate I had been working lately I would, indeed, be old very quickly.

"Well, you are younger than the old guy you replaced, aren't you? That makes you the young doctor in my book. Can't see why you want to argue the point."

"Yes, of course, of course, you're right" I answered, definitely not wishing to argue the point at two o'clock in the morning. "But, did you call to discuss my age or your emergency?"

"My God," exclaimed Mr. Yakobovitch. "Such a foolish young doctor. Of course I called to discuss my cow, not your age!" I was not pleased with how the conversation was going, but decided another retort would be counterproductive.

"Your cow?" I asked. "What's wrong with your cow?"

"Chavina just fainted, my young doctor. Imagine that. My biggest cow. She just calved a few days ago. She was fine, eating as usual. I just milked her a few hours ago. Everything was fine. Then this. She just keeled over. I think she must have had a stroke or a heart attack. She's breathing really rapidly and can't get up. I think she must be dying."

"No, no, Mr. Yakobovitch," I responded authoritatively. "She's got milk fever. I should be able to save her for you."

"But, she's got a normal temperature! What do you mean milk fever? I never heard of such a thing in Rumania and I had lots of cows there."

"But not like these cows, Yakobovitch! Anyway, I will explain it to you when I get there. I can't waste any time now. This is an emergency and I need to treat the cow right away."

"Say, young doc," interrupted Yakobovitch before I could hang up. "Do me another favor on your way out here. I have another emergency too. My wife, Anna, is sick too. Terrible diarrhea and vomiting. Would you stop by Dr. Hatzner's and bring him with you. It will save gasoline if you come together."

"Sure," I said. "Of course, I will stop by Hatzner's. It's right on the way."

"But if he's not there, or unable to come, you just come yourself! My cow needs you more than my wife needs Hatzner! Anyway, wives are easier to replace than good cows," he chuckled.

"OK, OK, Mr. Yakobovitch. Let me hang up and get started or you will for sure be replacing your cow!"

Twenty minutes later I was at Yakobovitch's place, without Dr. Hatzner who didn't answer his door because he was either an incredibly deep sleeper or out on another emergency. Despite the early hour, neighboring farmers had gathered around, all looking helplessly at the enormous cow lying on the ground with a huge, swollen udder.

"Yup. It's milk fever all right," I said authoritatively. A concerned murmur went through the crowd of onlookers.

"Yes, yes, but can you do something, young man?"

"Of course," I answered firmly. I went to my car and took out three bottles of calcium and my intravenous equipment and quickly returned to the cow. I got down on all fours, pressed on the cow's neck and injected the calcium directly into the jugular vein. It took all three bottles, but at the end of the third bottle, the cow suddenly turned around, lifted her head and then, to the amazement of everyone but me, stood up without difficulty, moved over to her trough and started eating as if nothing had been wrong.

"It's like magic!" exclaimed Yakobovitch. "I've never seen anything like it. You new young doctors sure know all the tricks! I'll bet old Doc Fertig couldn't have done as well!" Instantly my dislike of the phrase "young doctor" disappeared. I grinned from ear to ear, delighted with the compliment, although I knew full well that Fertig would have done exactly as I had and with exactly the same results. Actually, milk fever was quite common in Israel because of the intensive breeding for high milk production. The fact that it was considerably less common in Rumania and, therefore, generally unknown to most Rumanian immigrant farmers, was just a bit of luck which helped to build my reputation as a terrific vet!

"Hey, young Doctor," exclaimed Yakobovitch. "You did such a good job on Chaviva, why not come to the house and see if you can do something for my wife. There isn't too much difference, you know!"

Despite this last remark, I could tell he was serious. "Oh, no, sir!" I replied quickly, thinking back to the results of my "medical doctor" escapade in Ashkelon. "Even if I could cure her, which in this case I doubt, MDs are mean, you know! They don't like anyone intruding in their territory! I know from experience."

"I guess you're right, doc. I don't want you to get into any trouble anyway. Who would be there to take care of my cows when they need it?"

"Speaking of cows, here's how to take care of Chaviva so that she will not have this problem again. You have got to be careful with her because she has so much milk. It lowers her calcium level, and if you let it get too low, she will be back on the floor again. So, milk her a lot, four or five times a day, but in small amounts. Add a little calcium to her diet, and don't let her drink too much water at one time. Follow these rules, and she'll be fine."

Well, Yakobovitch never stopped talking about how I saved his cow from certain death. As he was the current president of the Farmers Council, his comments spread throughout the area and helped build my reputation among the private farmers.

Another event which helped was my "inside surgery" on Rachamim's cow. Most cattle in Israel were of the small local breed, not much good for meat, but extremely resistant to local diseases and well adapted to climatic conditions. The government had imported Brahma, Black Angus and Hereford bulls for breeding purposes to improve the quality of cattle for production of meat. Now, Rachamim was a Yemenite farmer with only one, small indigenous cow. He dreamed of having a big herd of cattle for the production of meat. After consulting with his friends, who had bigger and better herds than he, he decided that the first step to improve his stock should consist in breeding his one cow with an imported bull.

"So, how does this work, Doc?" he asked me one morning when I had stopped by to check on a minor problem with his cow. "Can an individual farmer breed his cows with the bulls the government imports?"

"Sure, Rachamim," I responded. "You just tell the government advisor" — each village had at least one official advisor to help make farmers out of the immigrants — "that you want to breed your cow with a Hereford. That will be the best match for her. The advisor will order the semen for you from the insemination center in Be'er Tuviah."

"Don't I have to take the cow to the bull in Be'er Tuviah?"

"Oh, no, the inseminator will come to you. It's all done with a glass tube. The bull never sees the cow at all."

"What a crazy world," said Rachamim. "My poor cow Yafa won't even have fun once a year!" he grinned at me with a sly look. "But how much will all this cost me, Doc?" he asked as a typical frugal Yemenite.

"Oh, probably 20 pounds, but it is well worth it, Rachamim. The offspring will be twice as big as your present cow."

"Twice as big! Wow! What if we used the semen from one of those big hunch-backed Brahma bulls? Then I could have a calf four times as big for the same price, no?"

"No way, Rachamim!" I interjected quickly. "Your cow could never carry and deliver a calf that size. Follow my advice and stick to a Hereford for this project."

I left and went on my way, not giving Rachamim's plans another thought.

Months later I got an urgent call. "Doc, you've got to come right away. Yafa has been trying to calve for several hours. My wife and I have been trying to help her, but nothing works. My wife is a midwife and knows all about difficult births, but she hasn't been able to help at all. We really need you!"

"Of course, I'll come at once. This is the calf from the artificial insemination we discussed some time ago?"

"Yes, yes. That's right. I'm very excited about it, too. It should be a big one."

When I arrived at Rachamim's barn, I could see that the cow was really having trouble. I quickly proceeded with a uterine inspection and found the calf was enormous and grossly deformed.

"Rachamim, what did you breed this cow with? It must have been a Brahma! There is no way that Yafa can deliver this calf. And the calf is so deformed in the head and neck, it's not even worth trying to save it. No point in putting Yafa through a Caesarean section. I'll do an embryotomy instead."

"Embryotomy? What's that?" asked Rachamim looking worried. "It means killing the calf and cutting it into pieces to allow it to pass through the birth canal," I replied as I reached for my special instruments for this procedure.

"Kill the calf? While it is still inside Yafa, *Adon Rofe* [doctor]? Can this be done? Is it safe for Yafa?" Rachamim and his wife both looked horrified.

"It will be a lot easier on her than a Caesarean, but it is still very difficult," I responded gravely. "I will be as careful as I can, of course. You should have listened to me when I told you not to breed her with anything but a Hereford! Now you may lose both the calf and the mother."

"*Yerachem Hashem* [God will have mercy]," responded Rachamim.

And he did. Within an hour the surgery was concluded. The barn looked like a butcher shop and I was covered with blood. But Yafa survived and would be able to be bred again soon.

"She's fine, Rachamim. You'll even have milk for awhile! Just be sure the next time you breed her it's with a Hereford!"

TALES OF AN UNORTHODOX VETERINARIAN   183

"Don't worry!" he replied earnestly. *"Temonim* [Yemenites] don't make the same mistake twice, *Adon Rofe!* But who would believe that such a surgery could be done without killing the mother, too! I wouldn't have believed it if I hadn't seen it with my own eyes! Surgery inside the cow. Imagine! You did a wonderful job!"

I smiled, remembering my first such surgery, with the two-headed calf in Migliarino. Back then I didn't even know the name of the procedure! This time I had the right tools and I knew what I was doing! I felt proud of my expertise and how far I had come since those days in Italy. It pleased me no end that Rachamim swore he would tell everyone in Gedera about my amazing "inside surgery" — which he did!

Building a reputation with the kibbutzim was a little tougher. There were no easy "miracles" to get me started! But, gradually, through lots of hard work and the introduction of a new government program to help combat mastitis, we achieved close to miraculous increases in milk production by the local herds.

My first big success was at Kibbutz Chazor. This was one of the two "American" kibbutzim in Israel. Ninety percent of it's members were Americans, mostly idealist refugees from the asphalt jungles of Los Angeles and other American cities, dreaming of a more pastoral existence in Israel. But the dream had a definite American flavor. In contrast to Kibbutz Nezach Yisrael, where the members all were dressed in traditional Jewish garb including sidelocks, black hats, and long *talish* tassels dangling from the waist bands of their work pants, Kibbutz Chazor was like a little slice of Texas. Everyone wore jeans and high-heeled cowboy boots and big Texas style hats. The barnyard was set up in the style used throughout Israel: long straight rows of stalls on either side of a covered passageway where tractors could pull in with big platforms of food to be thrown in the feeding troughs. But the entrance to the medicine room and manager's office in the barn had no *mezuzah* and there were no "with the help of God" inscriptions posted on every wall. Instead, Joey, the barn manager of Kibbutz Chazor, had covered his office walls with big posters of scores of Texas longhorns being herded by genuine American cowboys under the banner "Welcome to Longhorn Country."

The Kibbutz Chazor pastoral dream also included television. Although the members came to Israel seeking escape from American life, there was more than one element of America they couldn't give up. Television was one of them. So, there was one set in Joey's office, one in the big dining hall, and several others throughout the kibbutz, despite the fact that the only signal in the region came from Jordan and the few times you could receive a picture it would jump up and down more often than the belly dancer being broadcast on the screen.

Largely because of Joey, I decided that Kibbutz Chazor would be a good prospect for the government's new program to study and reduce mastitis. The program involved extensive use of antibiotics, which were squeezed into the cows' udders by hand using a special tube, a scrupulous regime of cleanliness while milking, education in the proper use of milking machines, follow-up analysis of the milk for bacteria at the Beth-Dagon Veterinary Institute, changes in the type or quantity of antibiotics based on the analysis, more follow-up testing, etc. It was more a question of "elbow grease" and perseverance than anything else, but with the right commitment I was certain the results would be spectacular.

Joey had a scientific bent and the patience to keep meticulous records. He was fascinated by technology and modern medicine. I knew that neither idealism nor religion would get in the way of improving his herd's milk production! In fact Joey was delighted that I wanted to work with him and his kibbutz and jumped into the program with relish.

Two months into the program, I stopped at the kibbutz for one of my regular weekly visits. Joey was waiting for me outside the barn with his tiny Moroccan wife who seemed to follow him everywhere. Roni was Joey's second wife (the first having been left behind in Los Angeles when he decided to move to the promised land). She was in her ninth month of pregnancy.

"From the size of Roni's belly, that kid is practically as big as she is!"

"Yes, Doc," he answered proudly. "This baby will be as tall as I am, and as gorgeous as his mother!"

"And he will also be a great lover of cows, since Roni has spent practically every waking moment with you on this project!"

"Successful project, you should say, Doc. I notice almost ten percent reduction in mastitis in the herd already! Of course, we still have a few tough problems. For example, today I discovered that one of the biggest cows, Goldie, has a bloody mastitis. You will have to take a look."

We went into the spotless barn to check her out. The udder was hot. When I squeezed the tit, the milk stream was bloody and as curdy as yogurt.

"Who milked Goldie last night, Joey?"

"Oh, Jesus," said Joey in English, a typical American response. "Now I know what happened. I took Roni to the hospital with false labor pains. I let the new guy do the milking."

"Well, an injection should clear this up pretty quickly," I said. "It usually does with this type of mechanical mastitis. You know that you have to watch all your milkers like a hawk, Joey, until they learn the importance of the procedures we have established. This guy probably forgot to wash his hands, or the cups on the machine, and look at the mess we have today!"

"You are right, Doc. It won't happen again. This is going to be the best milk-producing herd in the region! You'll see."

The practical results of the research done on the cows at Kibbutz Chazor were translated into improved treatment of mastitis throughout the region. Even though the other barn managers in the Gedera area were never as zealous as Joey in preventing the causes of mastitis, they did learn the importance of educating their milkers and enforcing cleanliness. Soon there was a steady decline in the incidence of mastitis in the region. In addition, through the research project at Kibbutz Chazor, I gained much better information about the types of antibiotics that were best to use in particular cases, making treatment much more effective. My acceptance as a veterinarian was complete once word spread about the results of the program and my educational efforts.

I grew to love the people of Gedera. Following whatever job I had been called to do, my clients would invite me to sit and drink coffee, or to have lunch or supper. Neighbors would always gather on these occasions and there was wonderful conversation and camaraderie. The new immigrants would tell tales about their countries. They were all proud of their new home, of course, but despite the traumas which had brought most of them to Israel, many had immense nostalgia for their old homelands, and, especially, for old customs and ways of doing things.

When they complained about how hard life was in Israel, the old timers would always interrupt with stories of the early days of colonization in Palestine, before Israel was a state.

"You think it's difficult now?" said Jacob Reznick, a real old timer, one day when a group of us had gathered for coffee at the home of one of my clients. "Let me tell you about the beginning of Gedera." Jacob had come to Gedera just before the turn of the century, when there was still nothing but jackals, weeds and snakes.

"We started plowing fields with wooden plows pulled by mules. We planted all these eucalyptus trees you see now. There was nothing here! The French baron (Baron Rothschild) sent us instructors that spoke only French. They were supposed to teach us how to grow grapes and produce wine! What a joke. We had almost no usable water. There were lots of mosquitos and malaria, the language and cultural barriers between us and our instructors were incredible, and finally there were the Arab marauders who tore out at night what we had planted during the day and stole any equipment they could lay their hands on. Even today I can't figure out how we actually survived, but we did. Today you guys have it easy!"

"And you know who really has it easy, don't you?" interjected Dr. Hotzner who never missed a chance for a little friendly rivalry. "Dr. Sorokin here. He just cruises around all day in his big station wagon, schmoozing with the farmers, checking out the animals for two minutes and staying for hours to drink coffee and eat cookies!"

"You must be kidding," I replied. "I've never seen you down on all fours in the mud to treat one of your patients. You MDs are the ones who have it easy. Seems to me you only operate in sterile hospitals surrounded by beautiful nurses!"

"Let's face it," laughed Manasche, our host for this afternoon, "we've all got the most difficult life . . . just ask anyone of us!"

Shortly after this discussion, I was called by Ziv, a young farmer who had a big herd and was very modern in his approach to animal care. "One of my cows is trying to calve, Doctor. But she's having trouble. I think she's going to need a Caesarean."

I knew it must be very serious if Ziv had not been able to get the cow to calve with his own expertise. "I will be there right away, Ziv! You just get the area around the cow ready for me to do my job."

"Bring your boots, Doc. She's in the yard, and I can't move her! It's pretty muddy out there."

"Great," I said to myself thinking of my recent conversation with Hotzner. "A difficult birth, plus mud!"

Twenty minutes later I pulled my car into Ziv's yard. All the neighbors were gathered in a big circle around Goldie, the cow, who was lying down in a tremendously muddy area of the yard, obviously struggling to give birth.

I pulled on my big rubber boots and made my way over to the cow. Since she was down, there was no alternative but for me to get all the way down in the mud with her.

As soon as I reached into the birth canal I could tell the calf was in a breech position. It was big, too. Too big to try and turn at this stage of labor. "You're right, Ziv. It will have to be a Caesarean. I guess we will have to do it out here, too. We can't move her now."

I looked around at the muddy area trying to figure out how to set the surgery up. "Ziv, get your tractor and pull over that wooden platform you've got stacked with wood over there. But take the wood off first," I called after him as he started for the barn. The neighbors helped unload the wood and tie the platform up to the tractor.

Meanwhile I squished back through the mud to my car to get the sterile instruments I would need. Storm clouds were gathering in the sky and a few raindrops fell. "First mud, now rain!" I thought. This was definitely going to be a messy afternoon.

Ziv used the tractor to get the heavy platform as close to the cow's belly as he could and together we pushed it into final position. The mud oozed through the wooden slats as I settled myself on the platform to lay out all my instruments. Once everything was ready, I gave Goldie an injection of a strong tranquilizer and began the surgery, down on my knees, mud still squirting through the slats as the platform shifted. The neighbors had moved back in a big circle again to watch from the fringes of the muddy area, but most of them wandered back to the shelter of the barn as the rain started to really come down. Ziv ran and got a tarpaulin, which he tried to hold over me during the surgery, but he was more in the way than helpful, and I shooed him away. Meanwhile, Goldie was an excellent patient. She didn't seem to mind the rain or the mud. Neither did her calf, which sprang into the muddy world on his own wobbly four feet almost as soon as I made the incision into Goldie's uterus. A cheer went up from the watching crowd!

Suddenly a loud voice called from the fence by the road. "Are you crazy, Sorokin, doing surgery out in the mud and in this rainstorm? If the cow doesn't die, you will certainly get pneumonia!" It was Dr. Hotzner, standing at the fence in his boots and stylish raincoat under a big shiny umbrella.

"Ah, just as I told you, Hotzner!" I laughed. "We vets really are made of stronger stuff than you MDs. And our patients are stronger than yours too. Look at this calf walking around! Why, it takes years for one of your babies to match that. Anyway, maybe now you will retract some of those comments you made about the easy job we vets have. I would like to know when was the last time you had to do surgery under such conditions!"

"OK, OK," he smiled, shaking his head. "I guess you earned your cookies and coffee today!"

I quickly finished up with Goldie. A short time later, she was back on her feet and nudging her wobbly calf toward the barn. I was covered with mud and soaking wet. "You certainly could use a shower and a cup of coffee, Doc. Come on up to the house and we will fix you up." Everybody, even Dr. Hotzner, followed us up to the house where, after I cleaned up, the conversation again flowed as freely as the Turkish coffee.

It was late when I returned home that night. "What have you been doing all this time," cried my wife as I walked in. "Dr. Schturman has called you five times!"

"Five times? What could that be about?" I wondered aloud. We looked at each other silently. We both knew in our hearts that, as it was close to ten months since we came to Gedera, there was a good chance the call would be about a new assignment. I put off returning the call until the next day, trying to delay the inevitable.

"Well, Dr. Sorokin," said Schturman when I finally called, "Dr. Fertig is returning in four weeks. We will have a new assignment for you, but I don't know yet where it will be. Just wanted to give you a little advance notice this time, since we gave you such short notice when we shipped you to Gedera! By the way, I understand things have gone pretty well there in Dr. Fertig's absence. Specially your work on mastitis has been excellent."

"Thank you, Dr. Schturman," I replied, pleased with the compliment, but saddened by the thought of leaving Gedera. I really hated to leave the practice and the people.

As I made my rounds that day I let everyone know that Dr. Fertig was returning in a month, and that we would be leaving. It was gratifying to see that my clients were genuinely sorry that I would have to move on. "We think you're great, Doc. Isn't there enough work for two veterinarians in this region? Maybe we should call the Hachaklait headquarters and tell them to let you stay! Dr. Fertig is getting old after all. You really accomplished more than he ever did anyway."

"Oh, no!" I responded quickly. "I appreciate the thought, but please don't call the Hachaklait. Don't do that!" I recalled Dr. Schturman's words when he sent me to Gedera: "Remember, my fine Italian doctor, we expect you not only to do a good veterinary job, but also to keep from criticizing your elders. And no showing off, if you know what's good for you!" I knew that any requests by any client for my continued presence would be somehow misconstrued and interpreted as a put up job, as criticism of my elders, and definitely as showing off!

Two weeks later I was summoned to the Hachaklait office to be given my new assignment. Dr. Schturman's desk was still cluttered. As he greeted me, he reached for a pile of papers in the center of the desk. "And what do you think this is, my fine Italian doctor?" I took a deep breath, knowing I was in for trouble, but without knowing what it could be. I shrugged and shook my head. "Letters from the farmers in the Gedera region. Everyone of them extolling your virtues as a veterinarian and asking for your assignment there to continue. Did you encourage this? Don't answer," he continued quickly as I started to protest. "You must have! Well, it certainly puts Dr. Fertig to shame. He is going to have to start all over again with his own clients when he returns! Imagine. Remember I told you you were there to help out, not to take over!"

"But, I didn't have any idea. . . .," I started to explain.

"Never mind, never mind," interrupted Schturman. "What's done is done. And anyway, you have proved yourself a good vet. You are ready for your own fulltime assignment, in Rosh Pina."

"Rosh Pina!" I exclaimed. "Is this banishment?" Rosh Pina was the northern-most region, isolated, and quite far from all our friends and relatives.

"Don't be silly," said Schturman. "But at least you will be far enough so that it will take some time for news of your shenanigans to reach us here at headquarters!"

I left the office with mixed feelings. I was thrilled to finally have a region of my own. Despite Dr. Schturman's protestations, however, I knew I really was being exiled. And all this for doing a good job!

Still, I was determined to make the best of it and when we left for Rosh Pina two weeks later, we decorated the car like newlyweds, with streamers and a big sign that said "Rosh Pina, Here We Come!" All the neighbors and many of my clients came to see us off and wish us well in the new assignment. The excitement was infectious. I soon forgot Schturman and the thought of exile and turned my future plans to conquering Rosh Pina!

XX

Pigs in the Holy Land!

*

Although I came into my own as a vet during my stint in Gedera, I clearly did not fit the model of the ideal Hachaklait veterinarian. Consequently, I was frequently at odds with the head office and some of my fellow doctors. Though they all gave me ample credit for my veterinary skills, nevertheless my initiative, drive and outlook on life were different from those of many of my colleagues, and that became the source of the problems. Let me try to explain.

At the center of the agricultural base in Israel were the kibbutzim, but there were also lots of small individual farmers, like Rachamim, the Gedera farmer who bred his cow to the big Brahma bull. Most of these small farmers joined together into *moschavim,* cooperative organizations created to sell the farmers' livestock and crops. The Hachaklait was a not-for-profit HMO, similar in concept to the HMOs that exist now in the United States for human medicine. It was formed by the umbrella organizations of the kibbutzim and *moschavim* to provide veterinary care for their animals. Each farmer or kibbutz that belonged to these organizations paid a certain fee per year per animal in return for all necessary veterinary services and medicines and the Hachaklait also insured each animal for 80% of its value. Since there were practically no private veterinarians in Israel, the Hachaklait filled a great need and became an extremely important organization. The lack of competition, however, also made it easy for bureaucracy to flourish and for the men in charge of the organization to remain very set in their ways and to protect their friends.

Each Hachaklait veterinarian was assigned his own region, except for the new vets like myself who served as substitutes until a region became available. The size of these geographic areas was determined by the number of animals to be cared for within the area. All the company veterinarians were salaried and paid strictly according to the number of animals serviced, so there was no monetary incentive to excel. "Quality control" was based mainly on the number and nature of complaints from farmers and kibbutzim. Of course, this meant that everyone tried hard to keep the complaints down. It also meant that anyone who worked harder or had more initiative than everyone else was a threat to the tranquility of the system. This was particularly true of substitute vets. If the substitute was too good, the assigned veterinarian suffered by comparison when he returned to work.

I have to admit I was not very sensitive to this problem. I was determined to prove myself a good veterinarian and I was also certain that by working harder than everyone else, my contributions would be rewarded with an assignment to a big region of my own.

Dr. Schturman was hard working and honest, but he hated to deal with problems, particularly if they involved any of his old friends. No wonder he had difficulty with me! In practically every job he sent me to I rocked the boat. That's why I knew in my heart that I was being "exiled" to Rosh Pina. Not only was it far away so "news of any shenanigans" would take some time to get to Haifa, it was also a new region, created by dividing in two parts an old region which now had too many animals for one veterinarian to handle. By sending me to Rosh Pina there would be no invidious comparisons to deal with for Schturman. Besides, he had assigned Dr. Ruben to handle the other half of the divided region. Ruben was really the only other "go-getter" in service of the Hachaklait. Perhaps Schturman thought that his two "problem children" would destroy themselves while trying to outdo each other as veterinarians of neighboring regions! Fortunately, as it turned out, Dr. Ruben and I became the best of friends. Unfortunately, we still got into trouble!

Rosh Pina is located at the foot of a mountain in the region of Israel known as the Upper Galilee. Unlike in most of Israel, the valleys in this region are naturally green. Streams of various sizes run from the towering, barren mountains, cutting their way through the countryside to the Jordan river and on to Lake Kineret (the Sea of Galilee). This precious water enables a wide variety of vegetation to flourish.

We had a spectacular view of the snow-capped Hermon mountains from our new home. Based on the scenery alone, we could almost imagine we were in Switzerland. But there was no chance of missing the Middle Eastern flavor of the tiny community. It was one of the original colonies funded by the Barons de Rothschild and Hirsch at the beginning of the century. Most of the early inhabitants had died during the terrible epidemics of malaria which plagued the Upper Galilee until the swamps of the Hachula Lake were drained in the early 1950s. A large proportion of the villagers were third-generation descendants of the first inhabitants, a real rarity in Israel at the time. This gave the village a sense of tradition and permanence that was absent from most Israeli towns. Diverse European traditions had blended with Middle Eastern culture, creating a distinct way of life which had not been significantly influenced by new waves of immigration. Some of the original stone houses, high up on the mountainside, were still inhabited. The steep cobblestone streets made them difficult to reach except on foot or by horseback. Arabian horses, always with fancy and colorful saddles, were still a common means of transportation in Rosh Pina, and competed with cars and jeeps on the roads — picturesque, although a bit dangerous, especially at night on the dark roads.

I met Dr. Ruben very soon after we arrived. He stopped by our house unannounced, a common practice in Rosh Pina — calling ahead of time was unheard of in those days.

He was tall and very good-looking, with a distinctive goatee, and I could tell by the way he strode up the walk that he was full of energy. "Hope I'm not interrupting your Shabbat afternoon plans," he said after introducing himself. "I thought we should get to know each other, Sorokin. I have heard a lot about you through the grapevine! Seems we have a lot in common: we are enterprising, work hard, and drive Schturman crazy!" he laughed.

As we sat and talked the afternoon away, it turned out we had many other things in common as well. We were both born in Vienna and immigrated to Israel before the war. Our families had a long tradition of dedication to Zionism. We both loved politics and community service. Neither of us was religious. Both of us were idealists, but not impractically so. We both were devoted to veterinary medicine. Needless to say, we hit it off immediately.

"You will love it up here," he assured me. "You have lots of kibbutzim in the valley. It's a natural place for them because of the water and fertile land. You work hard for them and they'll treat you like a king! Interesting work, too. Lots of opportunity for people like you and me. . . ." he smiled enigmatically. "You'll see. Well, I'm off," he announced suddenly bouncing to his feet. "See you soon and good luck." And off he went just as quickly as he had arrived, and long before I had a chance to ask him what he meant about the "opportunities."

I found my new clients easy to deal with. They were obviously pleased that the region had been split and that their new vet would have more time for them. They were even more delighted when they discovered that I started my activities at seven o'clock in the morning and was willing to work well into the evening if necessary.

I had a wide variety of kibbutzim in my region, ranging from less affluent ones, located in the mountainous area of the Galilee, to the relatively wealthier ones in the valley. Their main income was derived from apple orchards, cotton fields, fish ponds, poultry and dairy farming. Even the poorer kibbutzim in the region had modern equipment for milking, feeding and farming.

My patients were mostly cows and their major medical problems were malaria, mastitis and infertility. Malaria, transmitted by ticks, was a particularly troublesome problem causing jaundice, loss of weight and appetite, abortions and, of course, stopping all milk production. The disease was so pervasive I quickly decided that, although prevention of malaria was not part of my official duties as a Hachaklait doctor, I should try to tackle the problem. After some investigation I found out that the Beth Dagon Institute was working on an experimental vaccine. I suggested to one of the researchers that we do a joint research project using the cattle of Kibbutz Amiad as they were among the most seriously affected by the disease. Amiad's dairy cows were generally free of the disease, but the cattle raised for meat production grazed in wetlands heavily infested with malaria-carrying ticks.

It was reasonably easy to convince Arik, the chief herdsman, to participate in the project, which involved the injection of the cattle with the experimental vaccine consisting of modified malaria microorganisms.

"The vaccine is supposed to help increase the resistance of the cattle to the real disease," I explained. "But, because it is experimental, we will have to check the treated animals daily, not only to track the effectiveness of the vaccine, but to catch and treat any side effects."

"So you'll be here everyday?" Arik asked. "That's wonderful. We need a lot of help with the dairy herd as well. We lost our experienced barn man last week. The new guy needs some training. Surely you could squeeze in a few minutes with him everyday when you come to check on the cattle."

So, as a result, I spent quite a bit of time at Kibbutz Amiad almost every day. And Dr. Ruben was right: before long I was treated like royalty. "Of course you'll stay for lunch in the VIP dining room," insisted Arik whenever my visits were remotely close to midday. "We have got a thick juicy steak just waiting for you!" (Definitely not the normal kibbutz fare! How could I pass it up?)

"Take this small milk jug of fresh cream home to your wife. We know she's a good cook and can use it. You do so much extra work for us, you can't refuse." Although of no real monetary value, these gestures of appreciation for my extra efforts made me feel wonderful and inspired me to work even harder.

Actually I received similar VIP treatment at almost every kibbutz in the region. Even for these "modern," well-supplied kibbutzim, life was an enormous struggle. Idealism was no substitute for knowledge and experience, and idealism was what they had most of. They were especially appreciative of anyone who took the time to help educate and train their ever-changing members. Technically, the role of educator wasn't part of the vet's job either, but it was essential in order to achieve real success with animal husbandry. The extra effort not only paid off in fewer medical problems, but it also increased job satisfaction. I was not just a doctor, but also a teacher, counselor and confidant for the members of the kibbutzim in my region.

As I got to know my clients better, I soon learned that a majority of the kibbutzim in the Rosh Pina region also raised pigs! Actually the raising of pigs in the region of the Sea of Galilee dated back to biblical times. The place where Jesus chased the (presumably diseased) pigs into the sea to drown was only a few miles away in Tabcha on the shores of the Sea of Galilee. Undaunted by biblical pressure, the Christian Arab farmers had continued to raise pigs in the area.

At first the Jewish settlers had shied away from the practice and, as the kibbutzim proliferated in the region, enterprising Arabs soon discovered a wonderful new free source of food for their pigs: the leftovers generated by the kibbutzim family-style "all you can eat" service of meals. Kibbutz members always seemed to take more than they could eat, and the leftovers were substantial. The kibbutzim kitchen workers were more than happy to let the Arab farmers collect the leftover table scraps and kitchen garbage for their pigs.

"So how did you get involved in raising pigs?" I asked one day when Zigmund, the barn man at Kibbutz Kfar Blum, had given me a tour of the facilities, including the pig pens.

"Well, you know we used to give all our table scraps to the Arabs for their pigs. Then, gradually, it dawned on us that there might be profitable business in raising pigs, as they could become an excellent source of meat for the kibbutz, and that the same kitchen leftovers being given to the Arab farmers could be put to use closer to home!"

"But you're located on Jewish National Fund land! How do you get away with it?" I asked Zigmund.

"Well, naturally the religious muckety-mucks are having a fit," he laughed. "But they aren't politically strong enough to do anything about it. Look around you. Almost all the non-religious kibbutzim in this area are raising pigs. Of course, your bosses in the Hachaklait are a different story. They won't cover our pigs at all! Why don't you try and fix that for us, Sorokin?"

"Me?" I laughed. "They don't want to hear from me on even non-controversial matters. If they thought I was calling about providing veterinary services to pigs on Jewish National Fund lands, they wouldn't even answer the phone!"

"Well, I guess we'll get by the way we always have, using techniques we learned from the Arabs, from books and from occasional new members who know something about pigs. Still, it would be nice to have real veterinary services for them. . . ."

It was enough to get me thinking, but I didn't see that there was much I could do. I even discussed it with Dr. Ruben, but neither of us came up with a solution.

The weeks flew by. Dr. Schturman's first visit to check up on me was uneventful.. He actually seemed pleased, although it might have been because of the wonderful food my wife prepared for him more than for the results of my veterinary efforts.

Shortly after his visit he telephoned unexpectedly. "Well, Sorokin, we need your help. The doctor from the Zafeth zone above you has to leave for Switzerland immediately for emergency medical treatment. We have no one to replace him. It's a small zone. We reduced it a few years ago because of the Doctor's health problems. We will double your salary if you will fill in for him while he's gone. We recognize that, even for you, this will be quite an increase in workload, even if just the extra driving required is considered."

Well, I knew it would be impolitic to turn Schturman down, and we needed the extra money. Besides, I thought it was a sign of approval that he even asked me at all. So I agreed.

"Thanks very much, Sorokin," said Schturman, expressing what for him was extreme gratitude.

Undoubtedly he would have been considerably less enthusiastic about my acceptance had he known that my very first call in the zone would be to treat a pig!

I was just on my way out the door early one morning when the phone rang. "That you, Dr. Sorokin? The replacement vet?" It was Hans, the old Yeke barn man at Kibbutz Menara. "We have a serious problem here. Our prize sow got caught on some wire fence during the night, God knows how, and she cut herself really badly. We can't stop the bleeding. You must come at once! If we lose her, we lose her whole new litter, too."

"You know I'm not supposed to treat pigs, Hans! The Hachaklait would go crazy!"

"But, Doc, this is an emergency. The sow is going to bleed to death!"

"Ok, ok," I said. We can't let that happen. I was planning to come to Menara this week on a get acquainted visit. I will just speed that up and take care of the pig at the same time."

Forty minutes or so later I was at Menara stitching up the sow. "This was a pretty nasty wound, Hans. She really must have struggled to get free and made it worse in the process. Anyway, she should be ok. Here's a prescription for some antibiotics. I don't want to use the Hachaklait's medicine for this job."

"God forbid," commented Hans drily. "Anyway, we appreciate your coming even though it's not your job. What do we owe you?"

"Oh, nothing. Absolutely nothing, forget it. If I took money from you I would be in real trouble!"

"Then how about taking one of the little piglets to take home then, Doc? You don't keep kosher do you? White meat [the Israeli expression for pork] is really tasty."

"No, no Hans," I replied, mindful of the fact that I was in another man's district and had to watch my step. "I did this just because I hate to see any animal suffer. I don't need anything. Besides, I told you I was planning to be up here anyway later in the week. You just gave me a reason to come a little earlier, that's all."

Unwittingly, however, Hans had given me a great idea. I could hardly wait to get home to call Dr. Ruben and get his reaction.

"Ruben, you were right about the opportunities here! And I think I have figured out a way to take advantage of one in a way which will make our clients happy and will not violate any Hachaklait rules!"

"This I've got to hear!" exclaimed Dr. Ruben.

"Remember that we have talked about the need for veterinary services for the pigs? Well, suppose we agree to provide those services on our own time and have the kibbutzim raise a few pigs for us in exchange? We will write prescriptions for any needed medicines and tell the kibbutzim what supplies to provide us with, without ever using Hachaklait drugs or supplies. The only things that might not be one hundred percent kosher. . . ."

"Other than the pigs," laughed Dr. Ruben.

". . . . would be the use of the car and gasoline paid for by the Hachaklait."

"We can solve that problem," exclaimed Dr. Ruben. "We just limit our practice on the pigs to times when we would already otherwise be at the kibbutz. It's perfect."

Practically the next day we were in business, each in our own regions. The arrangements worked wonderfully. We provided "after-hours" veterinary services for the pigs, helping to improve both the quality and quantity of pig production in the region, while the kibbutzim willingly raised our pigs along with theirs providing us with a source of extra cash as well as food.

I was extremely busy, what with two regions and the extra work from the malaria project and the pigs. But I was happy. Dr. Ruben and I had become good friends as well as colleagues. My clients were pleased with my work. My family, although unhappy that I was working so hard and was never around, was comfortable and well accepted in Rosh Pina.

For the most part my work was routine. There were, however, occasional dramatic exceptions. One Sabbath morning, just after sunrise, I received a call from Kibbutz Hagoshrim. This was a kibbutz in Dr. Ruben's region, but as he was down South visiting his family, I had agreed to substitute for him. "We've got a real problem, Doctor," explained the caller. "One I bet you have never seen before: one of our cows has impaled herself on a metal fence pole! The pole is almost all the way through her! She's oozing blood. She's a really good cow, but I don't know if we should try to save her or put her out of her misery."

"Let's try to save her," I answered immediately. "I will be there as quick as I can. In the meantime get two tractors — the kind with the big lifts in front that you use to move bales of hay — and some long chains."

When I arrived some thirty minutes later there was a big crowd of kibbutznikim waiting for me. The large black and white cow was still alive, still impaled, obviously in great pain and probably in shock. This was definitely not something I had been prepared to handle in veterinary school. Improvisation was clearly called for.

I first gave the cow four bottles of glucose intravenously to help strengthen her. "Now move those two tractors in position on either side of her," I shouted to two of the kibbutz workers. "Ok, now let's put the chains under the cow and attach the ends to the tractor lifts. Then raise the lifts slowly, together! Try and keep them both at the same speed and height!" We all watched in hushed silence as the chains under the cow were lifted slowly upward by the tractors, pulling the cow up and finally getting her free of the fence pole. A cheer went up as the chains were gradually lowered and the cow was once again safe on the ground. Miraculously the pole had not hit any vital organs. The cow was slightly dazed and shaken, but not otherwise severely injured. I decided not to close the wound so it would drain properly and I loaded the cow with antibiotics to fight infection.

"Looks like she'll be all right," I said to the barn man. "She was sure lucky, though. Another few inches one way or the other and she would have been done for. I never saw anything like it in my life, that's for sure! I bet Dr. Ruben will be sorry he missed it!"

"We'll be sure to tell him all about it, don't you worry. Especially the part about how you used the tractors! Never thought that would work!"

News of the "crucified cow," as she became known, indeed spread throughout Dr. Ruben's region and my own. It even made its way to Hachaklait headquarters. But instead of praise for a job well done, all I got were hostile questions about what I was doing in Ruben's territory when he was supposed to be on duty.

"You two are becoming much too chummy," warned Schturman on the phone. "Don't think we don't know about your enterprises, the two of you," he said in a menacing tone. "You better stick to your own Hachaklait business from now on!" The emphasis on "your own Hachaklait" was unmistakable.

"Whew, Ruben," I exclaimed when I called to tell him of my phone conversation with Schturman. "He was mad! I mean really mad. Something is eating him besides this little incident of my substituting for you."

"Maybe he's jealous that we have figured out how to take care of the pigs."

"Well, whatever, I sure didn't like the tone of his voice."

My concern was obviously justified as was evident when Schturman paid his next visit. He was all business and very cold. At each stop on my rounds he thoroughly quizzed the barn men or herdsmen about my services.

"So, Arik, I understand Dr. Sorokin is very busy protecting your cows from malaria," he began when we arrived at Kibbutz Amiad. "I certainly hope his success warrants the time it takes from his official responsibilities!"

"Well, of course," responded Arik. "We are very pleased with the results, and also with the doctor's willingness to spend the extra time with us for the experiment. Here, look at the charts. They clearly show the experiment is helping reduce the disease. And the doctor never neglects his other responsibilities here, that's for sure."

"Well, the time he spends here might be more effectively spent elsewhere, you know," responded Schturman grumpily. "Prevention of disease is the job of the government, after all."

"Hey, I think I should get a little credit for this work, Dr. Schturman," I somewhat rashly protested. "After all, by reducing the incidence of malaria, I also reduce the illnesses and deaths for which the Hachaklait has responsibility. I think you should be glad that one of your vets has the initiative and drive to work on major health problems like this."

I instantly regretted the speech as Schturman just found it another excuse to reiterate his "you are just a young veterinarian, you should respect your elders" speech.

At Kibbutz Ayelet Hashachar he insisted on questioning the barn man intently about the incidence of mastitis, which had increased recently because of a change in barn personnel: such changes always caused problems in the barn! It was a never ending battle to try and keep up with the training and supervision of new helpers. Schturman, however, was just interested in the number of cases. Without giving me or the barn man a chance to explain the real reason, he launched into a lecture on the importance of cleaning the milking machines and the cows' udders and maintaining the appropriate milking pressure, as if I had never explained those issues to the barn man and his helpers.

The rest of the day continued in the same pattern. Wherever we went, he found something to question or complain about. He even asked one barn man whether I drank wine a lot and whether it interfered with my ability to handle my duties! I was shocked, since I never drank wine at all except at Passover. I really wondered what he was up to.

"Well, Sorokin. I don't think things here are as under control as you would like me to believe. You better really concentrate on your duties from now on! I'll be back to check up on things soon!"

Not a word was said about the pigs, but I couldn't help wondering if that was not the real source of his irritation. There was obviously nothing wrong with my service to my clients. They had only praise for my work and seemed as puzzled as I by his hostile, questioning tone.

I decided that the next time he came for a visit I would enlist my wife's efforts. He adored her cooking! Maybe a nice brunch before we went on our rounds would put him into a better mood.

I didn't have long to wait. The very next month he called and announced he would be paying another visit.

My wife cooked for two days in advance. She prepared a real feast! Schturman was in seventh heaven. "Frau doctor, I cannot tell what a treat this was. You have outdone yourself. I hate to pull myself away to go to work. But duty calls, you know." She beamed at the compliments. I gave her a big hug, and whispered "great job" in her ear as we left.

Our first stop was a small kibbutz not too far from our home. The barn man, was effusive in his praise of my work. I was a little embarrassed, but Schturman seemed amused by it rather than upset.

✳ ✳ ✳

"So what have you paid this guy, Sorokin?" he laughed. I laughed back, hoping that things would continue to go as well as they seemed to be going then. But, it was not to be.

While we were still in the barn, one of the new members of the kibbutz came in and seeing me he shouted out, "Oh, Dr. Sorokin. I'm so glad you're here. I want to go over your instructions on the new feed mixture for the cows."

"So now you are an expert on feed mixtures, Sorokin? Is there nothing you don't mix yourself in?"

"But, he really is an expert," exclaimed the barn manager. "Why I think this new feed, plus his work with malaria prevention have helped increase the herd's fertility rate substantially."

"But this is a matter concerning the *madrichim* from the Jewish Agency, not the Hachaklait doctors!" exclaimed Schturman, immediately lapsing back into his bureaucratic ways.

"Yes, that's true," responded the kibbutznik. "But these madrichim are never around when you need them! And Dr. Sorokin is always here helping. Why he even helps out with our pigs!"

There it was, out in the open. From the absolute silence that followed his words, the poor new kibbutznik realized he must have said something dreadfully wrong.

Schturman gave me a long look and strode out of the barn. The barn manager followed quickly, trying to repair the damage as best he could.

"Dr. Schturman, please come to the dining room for coffee. You are such an important man. Many of our members would like to meet you."

Schturman hesitated, and then agreed. He put on a happier face as he entered the VIP dining room where steaming cups of thick black Turkish coffee awaited us. The conversation was a little forced, but gradually became more relaxed as Schturman began to hold forth on his favorite topic of the kibbutzim of yesteryear, how different they were, how enthusiastic, how modest in expectation, how idealistic. . . .

Finally, we rose to leave. I was relieved that Schturman seemed to have gotten over his anger about the pigs. As we got to the door, the assistant dairyman stopped me.

"Did you bring your milk can Dr. Sorokin?"

"No, we don't need any milk, Yosi, thanks."

"So, you get free milk here, huh?" Schturman immediately attacked. "You know that is against the rules!"

I didn't bother to respond. He was right, of course, it was technically against the rules, but Schturman knew perfectly well that, without exception, every Hachaklait doctor received small gifts of milk or cream from clients as a gesture of appreciation for good service.

"I have seen enough," he said as we headed for the car. "No need to go anywhere else today."

I knew what that meant. There was no need to go anywhere else because Schturman had finally found his infraction of Hachaklait rules.

We engaged in some very polite conversation, but mostly sat in silence as I drove Schturman back to his own car which was parked at our house. After he left, I told my wife "There's going to be real trouble this time. I know it!"

"What? Over a little bit of milk? I don't believe it!"

But I was right. The next morning I was summoned urgently to the Hachaklait main office in Haifa. Schturman's office looked just the same as it had on my very first visit there. The desk was completely covered with papers and books. He sat in the same old chair, too. Now, as then, my fate was in his hands.

"Well, Sorokin. You mix yourself in things that aren't your job, you raise pigs in some kind of unholy alliance with Dr. Ruben, and you abuse your position to get free milk from your clients. Working beyond the call of duty is no excuse for getting free milk. This is a serious violation of the rules!"

I started to protest. "But, what about the other doctors. You know everyone gets a little free milk, now and then."

"We are not talking about the others!" he shouted. "We are talking about you. This milk business and your other activities, after you have been warned time and time again to stick to your assigned responsibilities, has brought us to an intolerable situation.

"They're going to fire me!" I thought. The room started spinning before my eyes.

"But what about my work? My clients are all very happy. No one complains. You heard them yourself!" I knew I was talking too fast and that I wasn't really being listened to, but I couldn't help myself. I really loved my job. I couldn't believe what was happening.

"We are not talking about your skill as a veterinarian. We are talking about discipline and company policy. You can't seem to conform, Sorokin, and that leads to trouble!"

"So what do you want me to do? Quit?" I was having a hard time fighting back tears at this point.

"We want you to resign. We will pay you two months salary for every year of service as a form of severance, and in recognition of the extra work you did. That's fair, we think."

"Well, I will resign for three months salary for each year of service," I said quietly after some thought. "After all, it will take me some time to find another position. I may even have to leave the country to find something I want to do. You know that government service is not my cup of tea and there isn't much else to do in Israel."

"Ok, it's agreed," said Schturman. "We will cut you a check now." In a few short minutes, my career with the Hachaklait was over.

On my way out, Schturman called me back. His expression softened. "Don't worry, Sorokin. You'll be fine. You are just like a cat. You always land on all fours. I know it will be that way this time too."

At the time, I didn't believe him. And for a while, we really struggled. We moved to crowded, bustling Tel Aviv, leaving behind the beautiful mountains and quiet countryside of Rosh Pina. I took a few temporary jobs in meat inspection, but I hated the blood and agony of the animals. There really were no veterinary jobs in Israel for me. I started to look for alternatives in Europe. One day an ad caught my eye in one of the veterinary magazines: "Needed-Assistant Professor in Small Animal Surgery-Contact University of Zurich, Switzerland."

I wasn't sure I qualified, but I called anyway. "When can you come?" asked the Swiss professor. "I think your experience in Israel is valuable, even if you didn't deal much with small animal practice. We know Israel's veterinary standards are high. I'm sure we can use you, if you can be here in ten days! The semester is about to start!"

"Yes, sir!" I exclaimed. "I'll be there!"

I was ecstatic. I was packed and ready to go within two days. Because I needed to leave immediately, we decided that my wife and children would remain in Israel until I got settled. They sent me off with tears and kisses at the airport.

As the plane soared into the air, I looked back toward Israel with a pang of sadness, knowing I might never return. The land disappeared. I stared at the white caps of the Mediterranean waves and finally sat back in my seat to dream about my new job, a new country, and a new beginning.

Epilogue

*

Animals have been a source of love, joy and amazement to me all my life, as well as a source of economic support. I shall always be grateful for the opportunities my life as a veterinarian has provided. In particular, I have enjoyed the marvelous range of interaction between man and other animals. I hope these stories of my early years in Israel, all of which are true, have provided you with a glimpse of the depth of that interaction. I also hope they have given you an understanding of the richness of the early formative years of the nation of Israel. Although I never returned to Israel to live, I still cherish it as my home, my country, and the homeland of my people. My memories of my life in Israel are as indelibly etched in my heart as the memory of my beloved Minka.